Myelodysplastic Syndromes

Editor

DAVID P. STEENSMA

HEMATOLOGY/ONCOLOGY CLINICS OF NORTH AMERICA

www.hemonc.theclinics.com

Consulting Editors
GEORGE P. CANELLOS
EDWARD J. BENZ Jr

April 2020 • Volume 34 • Number 2

ELSEVIER

1600 John F. Kennedy Boulevard • Suite 1800 • Philadelphia, Pennsylvania, 19103-2899

http://www.theclinics.com

HEMATOLOGY/ONCOLOGY CLINICS OF NORTH AMERICA Volume 34, Number 2
April 2020 ISSN 0889-8588, ISBN 13: 978-0-323-72259-9

Editor: Stacy Eastman
Developmental Editor: Kristen Helm

Photocopying
Single photocopies of single articles may be made for personal use as allowed by national copyright laws. Permission of the Publisher and payment of a fee is required for all other photocopying, including multiple or systematic copying, copying for advertising or promotional purposes, resale, and all forms of document delivery. Special rates are available for educational institutions that wish to make photocopies for non-profit educational classroom use. For information on how to seek permission visit www.elsevier.com/permissions or call: (+44) 1865 843830 (UK)/(+1) 215 239 3804 (USA).

Derivative Works
Subscribers may reproduce tables of contents or prepare lists of articles including abstracts for internal circulation within their institutions. Permission of the Publisher is required for resale or distribution outside the institution. Permission of the Publisher is required for all other derivative works, including compilations and translations (please consult www.elsevier.com/permissions).

Electronic Storage or Usage
Permission of the Publisher is required to store or use electronically any material contained in this periodical, including any article or part of an article (please consult www.elsevier.com/permissions). Except as outlined above, no part of this publication may be reproduced, stored in a retrieval system or transmitted in any form or by any means, electronic, mechanical, photocopying, recording or otherwise, without prior written permission of the Publisher.

Notice
No responsibility is assumed by the Publisher for any injury and/or damage to persons or property as a matter of products liability, negligence or otherwise, or from any use or operation of any methods, products, instructions or ideas contained in the material herein. Because of rapid advances in the medical sciences, in particular, independent verification of diagnoses and drug dosages should be made.

Although all advertising material is expected to conform to ethical (medical) standards, inclusion in this publication does not constitute a guarantee or endorsement of the quality or value of such product or of the claims made of it by its manufacturer.

Hematology/Oncology Clinics (ISSN 0889-8588) is published bimonthly by Elsevier Inc., 360 Park Avenue South, New York, NY 10010-1710. Months of issue are February, April, June, August, October, and December. Business and Editorial Offices: 1600 John F. Kennedy Blvd., Ste. 1800, Philadelphia, PA 19103—2899. Customer Service Office: 3251 Riverport Lane, Maryland Heights, MO 63043. Periodicals postage paid at New York, NY and at additional mailing offices. Subscription prices are $443.00 per year (domestic individuals), $876.00 per year (domestic institutions), $100.00 per year (domestic students/residents), $480.00 per year (Canadian individuals), $100.00 per year (Canadian students/residents), $1085.00 per year (Canadian institutions) $547.00 per year (international individuals), $1085.00 per year (international institutions), and $255.00 per year (international students/residents). International air speed delivery is included in all *Clinics* subscription prices. All prices are subject to change without notice. **POSTMASTER:** Send address changes to *Hematology/Oncology Clinics of North America*, Elsevier Health Sciences Division, Subscription Customer Service, 3251 Riverport Lane, Maryland Heights, MO 63043. Customer Service (orders, claims, online, change of address): Elsevier Health Sciences Division, Subscription **Customer Service, 3251 Riverport Lane, Maryland Heights, MO 63043. Tel: 1-800-654-2452 (U.S. and Canada); 314-447-8871 (outside U.S. and Canada). Fax: 314-447-8029. E-mail: journalscustomerservice-usa@elsevier.com (for print support); journalsonlinesupport-usa@elsevier.com (for online support).**

Reprints. For copies of 100 or more, of articles in this publication, please contact the Commercial Reprints Department, Elsevier Inc., 360 Park Avenue South, New York, New York 10010-1710; Tel.: 212-633-3874, Fax: 212-633-3820, E-mail: reprints@elsevier.com.

Hematology/Oncology Clinics of North America is covered in *MEDLINE/PubMed (Index Medicus), EMBASE/ Excerpta Medica, and BIOSIS.*

Contributors

CONSULTING EDITORS

GEORGE P. CANELLOS, MD
William Rosenberg Professor of Medicine, Department of Medical Oncology, Dana-Farber Cancer Institute, Boston, Massachusetts, USA

EDWARD J. BENZ Jr, MD
Professor, Pediatrics, Richard and Susan Smith Professor, Medicine, Professor, Genetics, Harvard Medical School, President and CEO Emeritus, Office of the President, Dana-Farber Cancer Institute, Boston, Massachusetts, USA

EDITOR

DAVID P. STEENSMA, MD, FACP
Edward P. Evans Chair in MDS Research, Division of Hematological Malignancies, Department of Medical Oncology, Dana-Farber Cancer Institute, Associate Professor, Harvard Medical School, Boston, Massachusetts, USA

AUTHORS

JANE MARGRET ANDERSON
Department of Hematology and Oncology, Mays Cancer Center, UT Health San Antonio MD Anderson Cancer Center, San Antonio, Texas, USA

MICHAEL F. BERGER, PhD
Department of Pathology, Human Oncology and Pathogenesis Program, Marie-Josee and Henry R. Kravis Center for Molecular Oncology, Memorial Sloan Kettering Cancer Center, New York, New York, USA

KELLY L. BOLTON, MD, PhD
Department of Medicine, Leukemia Service, Center for Hematologic Malignancies, Memorial Sloan Kettering Cancer Center, New York, New York, USA

ANDREW M. BRUNNER, MD
Assistant Professor, Harvard Medical School, Massachusetts General Hospital, Boston, Massachusetts, USA

AMY E. DeZERN, MD, MHS
Division of Hematologic Malignancies, Sidney Kimmel Comprehensive Cancer Center, Johns Hopkins University School of Medicine, Baltimore, Maryland, USA

JACQUELINE S. GARCIA, MD
Instructor in Medicine, Dana-Farber Cancer Institute, Harvard Medical School, Boston, Massachusetts, USA

JUAN GARZA, MD
Department of Hematology and Oncology, Mays Cancer Center, UT Health San Antonio MD Anderson Cancer Center, San Antonio, Texas, USA

NORBERT GATTERMANN, MD
Professor, Department of Hematology, Oncology and Clinical Immunology, Heinrich Heine University Düsseldorf, Düsseldorf, Germany

ARISTOTELES GIAGOUNIDIS, MD
Professor of Internal Medicine, Chair of Department of Hematology, Oncology and Palliative Medicine, Marien Hospital Düsseldorf, Düsseldorf, Germany

DIPTI GUPTA, MD, MPH
Department of Medicine, Cardiology Service, Memorial Sloan Kettering Cancer Center, New York, New York, USA

SABINE HAASE, CLS
Biomedical Analytics Specialist in Hematology, Department of Hematology, Oncology and Palliative Medicine, Marien Hospital Düsseldorf, Düsseldorf, Germany

ANTHONY M. HUNTER, MD
Malignant Hematology, Moffitt Cancer Center, University of South Florida, Morsani College of Medicine, Tampa, Florida, USA

RAMI S. KOMROKJI, MD
Senior Member and Professor of Oncologic Sciences, Section Head, Leukemia and MDS, Vice Chair, Malignant Hematology Department, Moffitt Cancer Center, Tampa, Florida, USA

ROSS L. LEVINE, MD
Department of Medicine, Leukemia Service, Center for Hematologic Malignancies, Human Oncology and Pathogenesis Program, Memorial Sloan Kettering Cancer Center, New York, New York, USA

ABHISHEK A. MANGAONKAR, MBBS
Assistant Professor of Medicine and Oncology, Division of Hematology, Department of Medicine, Mayo Clinic, Rochester, Minnesota, USA

AZIZ NAZHA, MD
Associate Staff, Department of Hematology and Medical Oncology, Director, Cleveland Clinic, Center for Clinical Artificial Intelligence, Assistant Professor, Cleveland Clinic Lerner College of Medicine, Case Western Reserve University, Taussig Cancer Institute, Cleveland, Ohio, USA

ELLI PAPAEMMANUIL, PhD
Department of Epidemiology and Biostatistics, Center for Hematologic Malignancies, Memorial Sloan Kettering Cancer Center, New York, New York, USA

MINAL PATEL, MPH
Center for Hematologic Malignancies, Memorial Sloan Kettering Cancer Center, New York, New York, USA

MRINAL M. PATNAIK, MD
Associate Professor of Medicine and Oncology, Division of Hematology, Department of Medicine, Mayo Clinic, Rochester, Minnesota, USA

RYAN N. PTASHKIN, MS
Department of Pathology, Memorial Sloan Kettering Cancer Center, New York, New York, USA

DAVID A. SALLMAN, MD
Assistant Professor, Malignant Hematology, Moffitt Cancer Center, Tampa, Florida, USA

ROBYN M. SCHERBER, MD, MPH
Assistant Professor of Medicine, Department of Hematology and Oncology, Mays Cancer Center, UT Health San Antonio MD Anderson Cancer Center, San Antonio, Texas, USA

KRISTEN E. SCHRATZ, MD
Division of Pediatric Oncology, Sidney Kimmel Comprehensive Cancer Center, Johns Hopkins University School of Medicine, Baltimore, Maryland, USA

JACOB SHREVE, MD, MS
Department of Hematology and Medical Oncology, Cleveland Clinic, Taussig Cancer Center, Cleveland, Ohio, USA

ROBERT SIDLOW, MD, MBA
Department of Medicine, General Internal Medicine Service, Memorial Sloan Kettering Cancer Center, New York, New York, USA

DAVID P. STEENSMA, MD, FACP
Edward P. Evans Chair in MDS Research, Division of Hematological Malignancies, Department of Medical Oncology, Dana-Farber Cancer Institute, Associate Professor, Harvard Medical School, Boston, Massachusetts, USA

ERIC S. WINER, MD
Adult Leukemia Program, Department of Medical Oncology, Dana-Farber Cancer Institute, Boston, Massachusetts, USA

AHMET ZEHIR, PhD
Department of Pathology, Memorial Sloan Kettering Cancer Center, New York, New York, USA

Contents

The recognition of cytologic dysplasia in blood and bone marrow remains the cornerstone of myelodysplastic syndromes (MDS) diagnosis because it distinguishes MDS from clonal hematopoiesis of indeterminate potential or clonal cytopenia of undetermined significance. Expert morphologists achieve high concordance in the diagnosis of MDS if appropriate clinical information is provided. Because of the low prevalence of MDS, diagnostic approaches based solely on molecular diagnosis will likely be erroneous.

Myelodysplastic syndromes (MDS) are a heterogeneous group of marrow failure disorders that primarily affect older persons but also occur at a lower frequency in children and young adults. There is increasing recognition of an inherited predisposition to MDS as well as other myeloid malignancies for patients of all ages. Germline predisposition to MDS can occur as part of a syndrome or sporadic disease. The timely diagnosis of an underlying genetic predisposition in the setting of MDS is important. This article delineates germline genetic causes of MDS and provides a scaffold for the diagnosis and management of patients in this context.

The acquisition of mutations in hematologic stem cells (clonal hematopoiesis) is common with normal aging and can be identified as an incidental finding through clinical genetic testing. Clonal hematopoiesis is associated with a heightened risk of developing hematologic neoplasms (especially myeloid) and accelerated atherosclerotic cardiovascular disease. This article discusses a multidisciplinary clinical approach to the management of patients with clonal hematopoiesis. Key areas of research needed to establish evidence-based clinical care guidelines and intervention strategies for individuals with clonal hematopoiesis are discussed.

Myelodysplastic syndromes are disorders of clonal myelopoiesis having a range of clinical manifestations, from benign and indolent to aggressive with very poor prognosis. Classifying the likely trajectory of disease within a patient largely guides therapeutic decision making and therefore survival. Traditional methods of risk-stratification systems rely on clinical features: simple blood tests, peripheral smears, bone marrow biopsies, and cytogenetics, but do not adequately predict disease severity for a substantial proportion of patients. This article reviews the state of stratification at use in the clinic, describes emerging systems that leverage large-scale genomic data, and summarizes efforts toward truly personalized prediction models.

Myelodysplastic syndromes are enriched for somatic mutations in the pre-mRNA splicing apparatus, with recurrent acquired mutations most commonly occurring in SF3B1, SRSF2, U2AF1, and ZRSR2. These mutations appear to be early events in the pathogenesis of disease, and, given their frequency and central role in leukemogenesis, are of interest as potential therapeutic targets. Clinical trials are exploring targets that directly affect the spliceosome (splicing modulators or protein arginine methyltransferase 5 inhibitors) or that exploit possible vulnerabilities created by alternative splicing (inhibiting ATR). Future research is needed to explore novel targets and therapeutic combinations and understand how these mutations lead to clonal dominance.

Anemia is the most common clinical manifestation of myelodysplastic syndrome (MDS), and most patients become red blood cell transfusion dependent. Defective erythropoiesis includes impaired terminal erythroid maturation. There are limited options for treatments of anemia in lower-risk MDS after failure of erythroid-stimulating agents. Luspatercept is an activin receptor type IIB fusion ligand trap novel agent. Luspatercept showed promising activity for treating anemia in patients with MDS with ring sideroblast subtypes. This article reviews the mechanism of impaired erythropoiesis in MDS. It summarizes clinical data with luspatercept and foresees how to best use this treatment in practice.

Sideroblastic anemias are a heterogeneous group of disorders unified by the presence of abnormal erythroid precursors with perinuclear mitochondrial iron deposition in the bone marrow. Based on etiology, they are classified into clonal and nonclonal. Clonal sideroblastic anemias refer to myeloid neoplasms with ring sideroblasts (RS) and frequently have somatic perturbations in the SF3B1 gene. Anemia is a major cause of morbidity in patients, and restoration of effective erythropoiesis is a major treatment goal. Morbidity includes transfusion and disease-related complications. This article focuses on treatment of acquired sideroblastic anemias and highlights areas of future investigation.

Mutations in *TP53* are observed in ~20% of patients with myelodysplastic syndromes (MDS), with increased frequency seen in patients with a complex karyotype and cases of therapy-related MDS. *TP53* mutations represent perhaps the single greatest negative prognostic indicator in MDS. Inferior outcomes are demonstrated with all approved treatment approaches, although hypomethylating agents remain the standard frontline treatment option. Although outcomes with allogeneic hematopoietic stem cell transplant are poor, it remains the only potentially curative therapy. Novel agents are required to improve outcomes in this molecular subgroup, with therapies that directly target the mutant protein and immunotherapies demonstrating greatest potential.

BCL-2 is an antiapoptotic protein that plays a critical role acute and chronic leukemias. Venetoclax is an orally selective BCL-2 inhibitor and BH3 mimetic approved in chronic lymphocytic leukemia and in combination with low dose cytarabine or hypomethylating agent in acute myeloid leukemia for the treatment of patients unfit for intensive chemotherapy. This article reviews the biology of BCL-2, focusing on its relationship to the myeloid microenvironment, and discusses the rationale for BCL-2 inhibition in myelodysplastic syndrome (MDS). Clinical trials testing venetoclax in MDS patients are under way. Potential biomarkers for clinical response to BCL-2 inhibition are discussed. Therapeutic opportunities for venetoclax in the therapeutic landscape of MDS are explored.

Secondary acute myeloid leukemia (sAML) is a complex diagnosis that includes AML caused by either an antecedent hematologic disease (AML-AHD) or from previous treatment with chemotherapy or radiation. This disease carries a poor prognosis and is historically chemorefractory; additionally, often patients are ineligible for standard chemotherapy because of advanced age and other comorbidities. The advances of molecular diagnostics and reclassification of World Health Organization criteria have aided in the categorization of this disease. This article describes the etiology and pathophysiology of sAML, and delves into past successful treatments as well as promising new treatments.

Iron overload (IOL) in patients with myelodysplastic syndromes (MDS) is mainly attributable to chronic transfusion therapy. The importance of iron chelation therapy (ICT) in MDS has been a matter of debate. The Telesto study, the only randomized, placebo-controlled trial of ICT with deferasirox in MDS, showed improved event-free survival with ICT in patients with lower-risk MDS. Although Telesto was not powered to detect differences between deferasirox and placebo for single-event categories of the composite primary endpoint for event-free survival, results are consistent with the view that iron-related cardiac dysfunction is ameliorated by ICT in elderly patients with MDS.

Myelodysplastic syndrome/myeloproliferative neoplasm overlap syndromes are rare types of chronic myeloid hematologic neoplasms. Patients with overlap syndrome have similar clinical features, mutations, and disease course, to other chronic myeloid malignancies. Limited data also suggests that overlap syndromes patients experience long standing and at times poorly controlled symptoms that may be underrecognized. In this article, we discuss the etiologies of symptoms in patients with overlap syndromes and currently available symptom burden assessment tools. Overall, symptom burden is an important consideration in patients with overlap syndrome, and efforts are ongoing to further investigate symptom burden and quality of life in this population.

HEMATOLOGY/ONCOLOGY
CLINICS OF NORTH AMERICA

SERIES OF RELATED INTEREST

Surgical Oncology Clinics of North America
https://www.surgonc.theclinics.com/

THE CLINICS ARE AVAILABLE ONLINE!
Access your subscription at:
www.theclinics.com

Erratum

For the article on "Radiation Therapy for Prostate Cancer" in the February 2020 issue of *Hematology/Oncology Clinics of North America* (Volume 34, Issue 1), a few errors occurred regarding the mentions of the Tables. On page 48, a mention of Table 1 was erroneously placed in the section, "Intermediate-Risk Disease". On page 51, a mention of Table 1 was erroneously placed in the section, "Definition and historical perspective". Also on page 51, at the end of the section, "Definition and historical perspective", the mention of Table 6 was incorrectly labeled as Table 7.

In the articles on "Radiation Therapy for Benign Disease: Arteriovenous Malformations, Desmoid Tumor, Dupuytren Contracture, Graves Ophthalmopathy, Gynecomastia, Heterotopic Ossification, Histiocytosis" and "Radiation Therapy for Benign Disease: Keloids, Macular Degeneration, Orbital Pseudotumor, Pterygium, Peyronie Disease, Trigeminal Neuralgia" in the same issue, the author, Lisa Jane Sudmeier, MD, was erroneously omitted from the author list.

The online version of this issue has been corrected.

hemonc.theclinics.com

Preface

Myelodysplastic Syndromes

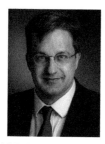

David P. Steensma, MD, FACP
Editor

The myelodysplastic syndromes (MDS) continue to place a heavy burden on affected patients and also deeply challenge the clinicians caring for those patients. Discovery of more than 50 recurrent MDS-associated somatic mutations, and improved understanding of numerous other aspects of disease pathobiology, has not yet led to approval of any targeted precision medications for MDS. In fact, the precise mechanisms by which 2 of the 3 drugs approved by the Food and Drug Administration (FDA) for MDS-related indications lead to clinic benefit - azacitidine (approved more than 15 years ago, in 2004) and decitabine (approved 2006) - remain uncertain.

Still, not all is doom and gloom. The FDA approved 8 medications for treatment of acute myeloid leukemia (AML) in 2017 to 2018, and it is likely that at least several of these will be useful for subsets of MDS patients. A growing understanding of clonal hematopoiesis and the mechanisms by which this extremely common proinflammatory malignancy precursor state evolves, identification of a growing roster of germline mutations that predispose to MDS, and refining of prognostic models hint of major changes to come. Perhaps someday it will even be possible to prevent MDS development and progression in at-risk persons.

In this issue of *Hematology/Oncology Clinics of North America* focused on MDS, 12 groups of experts have provided concise summaries and perspectives on areas of current interest and challenge within this group of diseases. These challenges begin with diagnosis; Giagounidis reviews the continued role of traditional morphology in the era of widely available DNA sequencing panels, while Schratz and DeZern tackle the difficulty of interpreting results of those panels and distinguishing somatic from germline variants. Bolton and her colleagues discuss the clinic that they have created to evaluate and counsel patients with clonal hematopoiesis, while Shreve and Nazha summarize recent developments in prognostic modeling.

Somatic mutations in genes encoding core components of the spliceosome are the most common class of mutation in MDS; Brunner and I review prospects for splicing-

Hematol Oncol Clin N Am 34 (2020) xv–xvi
https://doi.org/10.1016/j.hoc.2019.12.001
0889-8588/20/© 2019 Published by Elsevier Inc.

targeted therapies. One of these recurrent splicing mutations, SF3B1, is strongly associated with MDS with ring sideroblasts, the group of disorders for which luspatercept showed improved hemoglobin and reduced transfusion needs in a randomized placebo-controlled trial; Komrokji reports on these developments. Mangaonkar and Patnaik provide a comprehensive overview of sideroblastic anemias more generally.

Patients with TP53 mutations are a very difficult group to help. They have a poor prognosis and tend to be refractory to traditional cytotoxic drugs, and relapse quickly after treatment with a DNA hypomethylating agent. Several new molecules in development focus on this major unmet need, as reviewed by Hunter and Sallman. Garcia discusses combination therapy with venetoclax, which has rapidly become a standard of care in older patients with AML and may also prove useful in MDS. Higher-risk mutations, such as TP53, are enriched in patients with secondary and therapy-related myeloid neoplasms, including secondary AML, as reviewed by Winer.

Iron chelation has historically been one of the more controversial areas of MDS practice. Gattermann reviews the pros and cons of chelation therapy in the context of the recent results of the long-awaited TELESTO randomized placebo-controlled trial of deferasirox. Finally, Garza and colleagues discuss the challenging group of syndromes in which MDS overlaps with myeloproliferative features with a particular focus on patient-reported outcomes and health-related quality of life.

I hope that readers will enjoy these summaries as much as I have and will find them useful.

David P. Steensma, MD, FACP
Division of Hematological Malignancies
Department of Medical Oncology
Dana Farber Cancer Institute
450 Brookline Avenue
Boston, MA 02215, USA

E-mail address:
david_steensma@dfci.harvard.edu

Where Does Morphology Fit in Myelodysplastic Syndrome Diagnosis in the Era of Molecular Testing?

Aristoteles Giagounidis, MD*, Sabine Haase, CLS

KEYWORDS

- Myelodysplastic syndromes • Morphology • Diagnosis • Algorithm

KEY POINTS

- The recognition of cytologic dysplasia in blood and bone marrow remains the cornerstone of myelodysplastic syndromes (MDS) diagnosis because it distinguishes MDS from clonal hematopoiesis of indeterminate potential or clonal cytopenia of undetermined significance.
- Expert morphologists achieve high concordance in the diagnosis of MDS if appropriate clinical information is provided.
- Because of the low prevalence of MDS, diagnostic approaches based solely on molecular diagnosis will likely be erroneous.

INTRODUCTION

Myelodysplastic syndromes (MDS) are heterogeneous myeloid disorders. This heterogeneity is evident not only in the broad range of cytogenetic or molecular abnormalities that have been described but also in the morphologic subtleties that exist in the myelodysplastic universe (**Table 1**). Myelodysplasia in the blood and bone marrow is far from being specific or pathognomonic for MDS, though. Dysplastic cell abnormalities have been reported in a panoply of benign and malignant diseases as well as in patients with metal poisoning or drug toxicity.[1–8] The morphologic diagnosis of MDS is further hampered by the fact that the number of clinicians training in MDS morphology is decreasing steadily in many countries, including Germany, France, the United Kingdom, and the United States (Marie-Thérèse Daniel, personal communication, 2010). However, integrating the clinical picture, patient history, family history, exposure to toxins, blood results as well as the signs and symptoms of the disease

Klinik für Hämatologie, Onkologie und Palliativmedizin, Marien Hospital Düsseldorf, Rochusstr. 2, Düsseldorf 40479, Germany
* Corresponding author.
E-mail address: aristoteles.giagounidis@vkkd-kliniken.de

Hematol Oncol Clin N Am 34 (2020) 321–331
https://doi.org/10.1016/j.hoc.2019.11.005
0889-8588/20/© 2019 Elsevier Inc. All rights reserved.

hemonc.theclinics.com

Table 1
Morphologic abnormalities occurring in myelodysplastic syndromes

Erythropoiesis	Granulopoiesis	Megakaryocytes
Megaloblastoid abnormalities	Degranulated precursors	Micromegakaryocytes
Irregular nuclear outline	Hyposegmentation	Mononuclear megakaryocytes
Multinuclearity	(pseudo-Pelger cells)	Multiple disparate
Karyorrhexis	Hypersegmentation	megakaryocytic nuclei
Internuclear bridging	Abnormal chromatin clumping	
Small nuclear fragments	Chromatin filaments	
Nuclear budding	Partial peroxidase deficiency	
Nuclear-cytoplasmic		
asynchrony		
Basophilic stippling		
Cytoplasmic vacuolization		
Ring sideroblasts		
PAS-positivity of erythroid		
precursors		

into the process of MDS diagnosis is of paramount importance because it increases the pretest probability to pinpoint the disease. Finally, it takes a considerable amount of time to reach expert level in bone marrow cytomorphology (**Table 2**). During this process, it is essential to recognize the optimal area of a smear for the enumeration of cells, the morphologic abnormalities that can be due to aging, to artifacts from suboptimal blood and bone marrow smear preparation, to changes in the pH of the stain used, as well as the statistical effect of counting a limited number of cells (**Table 3**). Carlo Aul, one of Germany's great cytomorphologists, coined the sentence: "People don't look enough at normal bone marrows," pointing to the fact that one needs to know what is normal before identifying the abnormal. Finally, even experts in cytomorphology need not necessarily agree on a given diagnosis. A study from Japan from 2018 regarding enumeration of blasts and the degree of dysplasia in MDS bone marrows showed substantial, albeit not perfect, correlation between expert morphologists.[9] There has been a shift in the diagnostics of MDS in the last decades. First, with the advent of flow cytometry, abnormalities on the cell surface were supposed to improve diagnostics and render morphology unnecessary. A laboratory consultant told one of the authors 20 years ago that "in a few years' time" morphology will be

Table 2
Morphologic diagnosis of myelodysplastic syndromes is dependent on experience

Number of Bone Marrow Slides You Have Examined	What You Can Expect
<100	You know where to switch on the microscope
100–300	No confidence[a]
300–900	Overconfidence[b]
>900	You are humbled
>1500	Experienced
>5000	Very experienced
>10,000	Expert

[a] You are making a lot of wrong diagnoses and you realize it.
[b] You are making a lot of wrong diagnoses and you do not realize it.

Table 3 Variation of cell counts according to cells enumerated	
Cell Count	Variability at ±2 Standard Deviations for a Hypothetical Cell Percentage of 20%
100	12–28
200	14.5–25.5
500	16.6–23.6
1000	17.6–22.5

Data from Rümke CL. [Confidence intervals]. Ned Tijdschr Geneeskd 1989;133(41):2013-2015.

taught in the institute of medical history rather than in pathology. However, the reality has turned out to be different. The same might be true for the promises of salvation attributed to molecular analysis. This article persuades the reader that cytomorphology and histopathology of blood and bone marrow will remain the linchpin of MDS diagnostics and are not yet to be substituted for by any of the new fancy analytics blatantly advertised. On the other hand, it also aims to show that the combination of morphologic and complementary analyses (including flow cytometry and genetic testing) will likely deliver the highest degree of diagnostic accuracy.

DIAGNOSTIC CONCEPT

The diagnostic concept of MDS requires the evidence of cytopenia, dysplasia in major myeloid cell lineages (erythroid, myeloid, megakaryocytic), and the proof of clonality.[10,11] The degree of cytopenia is ill defined, but from a conceptual point of view any degree of cytopenia would suffice.[12] Proof of clonality may be morphologic (ie, blast excess), cytogenetic, or molecular. However, cytogenetic or molecular abnormalities need not be specific for MDS: Loss of chromosome Y may happen in physiologic male senescence, and several mutations recurrently reported in MDS have also been described in apparently healthy individuals without evidence of cytopenia.[10] In an attempt to define minimal diagnostic criteria of MDS, an international working group went to great lengths to attribute different diagnostic weight to various parameters necessary for the diagnosis of MDS.[11] **Fig. 1** shows an algorithm according to those suggestions. The shaded areas all involve cytomorphology and underscore its importance in the ascertainment of MDS. Molecular abnormalities are only "cocriteria," unable to sustain a diagnosis of MDS without additional parameters. Whether it is correct to require 2 or more cocriteria, or to allow an MDS diagnosis solely on the basis of an abnormal karyotypic abnormality without evidence of morphologic dysplasia, warrants further discussion. For the diagnosis of MDS with excess blasts, myelodysplasia is not compulsory. Therefore, the algorithm puts the requirement of greater than 10% dysplastic cells in any myeloid cell lineage below that of other factors. On the other hand, in the case of bone marrow blasts of less than 5%, myelodysplasia, that is, morphologically abnormal blood cell maturation, remains a major distinctive criterion, putting cytomorphology in the front seat.

THE MOLECULAR ERA

More than 40 genes have been recognized as being recurrently mutated in patients with MDS.[13] SF3B1 and TET2 are common, being present in up to 25% of cases, whereas most other gene mutations are far less abundant in a single patient. Some

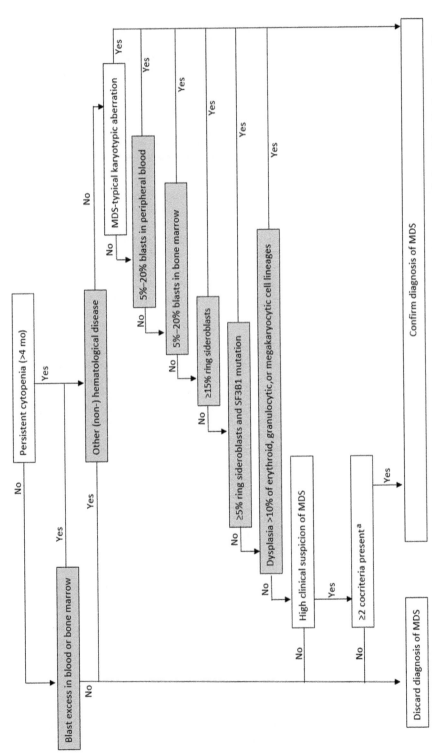

Fig. 1. MDS diagnosis according to International MDS Working Group Experts. Shaded rectangles involve cytomorphology. [a] Cocriteria: abnormal bone marrow histopathology supporting MDS, abnormal immunophenotyping supporting MDS, clonality of myeloid cells with MDS-typical molecular aberrations.

mutations, and the occurrence of multiple mutations, might herald a higher likelihood of MDS development if identified in healthy individuals (**Table 4**). It is logical, therefore, that molecular abnormalities have been integrated in the algorithm for the diagnosis of MDS, especially in equivocal cases. However, they are not the panacea, and several considerations come into play when the contribution of each method is carefully examined: Specificity of gene mutations, reliability of morphology, and additional investigations able to refine the diagnostic process.

SPECIFICITY OF GENE MUTATIONS: CHIP–CHOPping AROUND ICUS AND CCUS

The increasing availability of mutational analysis with next-generation sequencing (NGS) has made it possible to examine large numbers of healthy individuals as well as patient populations and has allowed us to group them into different categories. The first category might be taken as clinically irrelevant because the patient does not suffer from any objective blood abnormality. It is the recognition that there is significant clonal hematopoiesis (ie, >2% variant allele frequency), but no cytopenia, which is called clonal hematopoiesis of indeterminate potential (CHIP).[14] If the gene mutations are known to have "oncogenic potential," CHIP becomes CHOP (clonal hematopoiesis with oncogenic potential).[15] In both instances, morphology by definition is unable to reveal any abnormality. The other end of the spectrum is idiopathic cytopenia of undetermined significance (ICUS). Here, there is a patient with objective cytopenia. However, clonality has not been established. It could be any disease out of the nonclonal spectrum of **Fig. 2**, ethnic cytopenia, or a normal variant. Morphology again is noncontributory. Once clonality is established, these patients become clonal cytopenias of undetermined significance (CCUS). Here, morphology is of decisive importance, because CCUS excludes patients with significant dysplasia. Those would be called MDS. The diagnostic challenge in this pre-MDS universe is a relatively low prevalence of gene mutations, which leads to unacceptable low positive predictive values,

Table 4
Important genetic mutations in myelodysplastic syndromes patients

Function	Gene	Prognosis	Incidence, %
Epigenetic regulation	TET2	Unclear	25
	ASXL1	Unfavorable	20
	DNMT3A	Probably unfavorable	15
	EZH2	Unfavorable	7
	IDH	Unfavorable	3
Splicing genes	SF3B1	Favorable	30
	SRSF2	Unfavorable	15
	U2AF1	Unfavorable	10
	ZRSR2	Unfavorable	7
Transcription factors	RUNX1	Unfavorable	15
	TP53	Very unfavorable	10
	ETV6	Unfavorable	<5
Others	RAS	Unfavorable, more common in CMML	7
	STAG2	Unclear	5
	BCOR	Unfavorable	5

Data from Bejar R, Stevenson KE, Caughey B, et al. Somatic mutations predict poor outcome in patients with myelodysplastic syndrome after hematopoietic stem-cell transplantation. J Clin Oncol 2014;32(25):2691-2698.

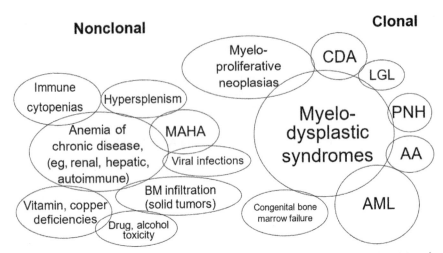

Fig. 2. Differential diagnosis of MDS. Clonal and nonclonal causes of cytopenias. AA, aplastic anemia; BM, bone marrow; CDA, congenital dyserythropoietic anemia; LGL, large granular lymphocytes; MAHA, microangiopathic hemolytic anemias; PNH, paroxysmal nocturnal hemoglobinuria.

and a high error rate of NGS reads owing to artifacts introduced during sample preparation and sequencing,[16] including amplification bias during polymerase chain reaction, polymerase mistakes, errors during sequencing cycles, and others.[17] Also, some point mutations may be difficult to distinguish from benign polymorphisms, and incidental passenger mutations that are unrelated to the disease may be considered driver mutations.[18] Although many clinicians intuitively understand that subtle abnormalities in morphology may go undetected to the less experienced cytomorphologist, they might not realize the intricate impact of prevalence of a mutation on reliability of a sequencing result.

DEPENDENCE OF NEXT-GENERATION SEQUENCING RESULTS ON PREVALENCE OF A MUTATION

Table 5 shows the prevalence of a given mutation in patients with MDS. If mutation analysis is extended to equivocal cases, and more so to a broader population, the probability of finding a mutation by NGS falls sharply, because most samples will not be MDS and therefore negative for the gene mutation sought. At a variant allele frequency of 1% in a single patient, an Illumina HiSeq2500 system will return a positive predictive value of 50%,[17] which means you can flip a coin whether the gene mutation

Table 5
Low prevalence of a disease reduces positive predictive value of a test

	Disease Present	Disease Absent	Positive Predictive Value	Negative Predictive Value
Test positive	20	100	20/120 = 17%	
Test negative	0	99.880		100%
	20	99.980		

is really present or not. Assume one screens an entire town with NGS sequencing. It is known that MDS has an overall prevalence of 20/100,000. If one screens 100,000 patients for MDS with a test that has a specificity of 99.9% and a sensitivity of 99.9%, the probability that a patient with a positive result will definitely have the MDS mutation is far from being 99.9%. It is 17% (see **Table 5**). With a sensitivity of 99.9%, the test is certainly going to identify the 20 true MDS patients. However, with a specificity of 99.9%, and a low prevalence of 20 in 100,000 patients, the test will produce 100 false positive results (0.1% of 100,000). Add those to the 20 correctly identified positive results and you end up with 120 positives, although only 20 have the disease. The positive predictive value of this test is going to be 20 divided by 120 (17%), which is unacceptable. To overcome this weakness (eg, of NGS in a disease with low prevalence), one can apply 2 methods: Increase sensitivity and specificity to 1×10^8 with duplex sequencing; this will be more time consuming and costly; or increase the pretest probability by examining only patients with a high probability of MDS, so that the false positives are lower. The best method to do this is going to apply a good medical history, review of peripheral blood counts, clinical examination, and expert blood and bone marrow morphology.

RELIABILITY OF MYELODYSPLASTIC SYNDROMES MORPHOLOGY

Although bone marrow cytomorphology may seem very subjective, the concordance of international reviewers in making a diagnosis is high. The German Competence Network "acute and chronic leukemias" funded a morphology review study with international experts reviewing bone marrow cytomorphology slides with attached clinical information. The reviewers are listed in **Table 6**. Slides were sent out twice. In the first round, bone marrow slides included MDS with multi-lineage dysplasia (MDS-MLD), megaloblastic anemia, del(5q) MDS, acute myeloid leukemia (AML), and a normal bone marrow smear (**Box 1**). In the second round, all slides were either early or advanced MDS, chronic myelomonocytic leukemia (CMML), or AML. As shown in **Table 3**, even when counting 500 cells, there remains a narrow confidence interval, which makes variations in the range of 2% possible. Accepting this "margin of error," the results of the reviewers gave an overall concordance of 97.5% in the first round and 92.5% in the second round. Even when applying very strict criteria (no "margin of error" accepted), round 1 would come up with a 90% concordance, whereas round 2 would yield 80% (**Tables 7** and **8**).

Table 6	
International reviewers of the German Competence Network "acute and chronic leukemia" cytomorphology review panel	
Barbara Bain	United Kingdom
John Bennett	United States
Winfried Gassmann	Germany
Ulrich Germing	Germany
Aristoteles Giagounidis	Germany
Jean Goasguen	France
Torsten Haferlach	Germany
H. A. Horst	Germany
Helmut Löffler	Germany
Teresa Vallespi	Spain

Listed in alphabetical order.

Box 1
Slides sent in the first blinded review round

1. Myelodysplastic syndromes with multilineage dysplasia

2. Megaloblastic anemia

3. del(5q) MDS

4. Acute monoblastic leukemia

5. Bone marrow of a healthy volunteer

Slides sent in the second review round:
1. Myelodysplastic syndromes with excess blasts-1
2. Pure erythroid leukemia (FAB M6a)
3. Chronic myelomonocytic leukemia 1
4. Low blast acute myeloid leukemia (previous RAEB-T)
5. Acute myeloid leukemia

EXCLUSION OF ALTERNATIVE DIAGNOSES

Several pathologic conditions may present with cytopenias that have evolved over a longer period of time. Several of those can be readily excluded by cytomorphology or histopathology, for example, hairy cell leukemia, splenic marginal zone lymphoma, aplastic anemia, bone marrow infiltration by solid tumors, and others.

WEAKNESS OF CYTOMORPHOLOGY

Teaching and being taught cytomorphology is a time-consuming activity. Although international experts might reach high agreement rates, your bone marrow cytomorphologist might not be an expert. This major weakness can only be overcome by central reviews of bone marrow smears and by intensifying the efforts in teaching. Another point is that morphologic abnormalities in a biological system like the human bone marrow show wide variabilities and are rarely pathognomonic. Apart from a substantial increase in blasts, which is never physiologic, most abnormalities can be seen in alternative diagnoses, hence the necessity to rule out another disease before attempting to make the diagnosis of MDS (see **Fig. 2**). Time constraints in daily work may lead to misdiagnosis, which underscores the necessity of thorough clinical review and the importance of providing the pathologist with as much clinical information as possible. Finally, certain abnormalities are ill defined, including blast

Table 7
Results of the reviewers in round 1

	1	2	3	4	5	6	7	8
MDS-MLD[a]	+	+	(+)	+	+	+	(+)	(+)
Megaloblastic anemia	+	+	+	+	+	+	+	+
del(5q) MDS	+	−	+	+	+	+	+	+
AML	+	+	+	+	+	+	+	+
Healthy	+	+	+	+	+	+	+	+

Reviewer numbers do not match the alphabetical order of reviewer names for data protection reasons. In each round, 1 reviewer did not return results.
[a] Five out of 8 reviewers diagnosed MDS-MLD; 3 reviewers diagnosed RAEB-1.

Table 8
Results of the reviewers in round 2

	1	2	3	4	5	6	7	8
MDS-EB1[a]	+	(+)	(+)	+	(+)	+	+	+
Pure erythroid leukemia	+	+	+	+	+	+	+	+
CMML-1[b]	+	−	+	+	+	+	+	(+)
RAEB-T	+	+	+	+	+	+	+	+
AML[c]	+	+	(+)	+	−	−	+	+

Reviewer numbers do not match the alphabetical order of reviewer names for data protection reasons. In each round, 1 reviewer did not return results.
[a] Two RAEB-2 and 1 MDS-MLD result.
[b] One result of reactive bone marrow changes, and one result of MDS-EB2.
[c] One result of MDS-EB1, one result of MDS/MPN, and one result of MDS-EB2.

morphology and ring sideroblasts, although numerous attempts have been made to standardize their diagnosis.[19] For example, blasts are usually defined as cells with high nuclear/cytoplasmic ratio, easily discernible nucleoli, and fine nuclear chromatin. The cytoplasm is narrow and usually devoid of granules, although type II myeloid blasts might contain a variable amount of azurophilic granulation. No Golgi zone is to be detected.[19] However, AML with t(8;21) translocation is the quintessential example displaying blasts with distinct Golgi zones (for examples, see ASH Image bank or Refs.[20,21]). For this reason, evaluation of bone marrow morphology of MDS cases must take into account individual variations, which complicates things further.

SO, WHERE DOES MORPHOLOGY FIT IN THE ERA OF MOLECULAR TESTING?

It is the authors' firm belief that morphology is still the cornerstone of MDS diagnosis. A molecular abnormality that has not translated into morphologic abnormality, that is, has not developed a phenotypic abnormality, is not (yet) a disease, and this is also what international conventions suggest. On the other hand, a clearly dysplastic bone marrow that couples with cytopenia will be called a disease, because scientific understanding is that morphologic abnormality leads to cytopenia and not vice versa. This holds true irrespective of the fact of whether there will be cytogenetic or molecular abnormalities. The current paradigm, therefore, which excludes MDS if there is no morphologic abnormality, should still hold true. Whether cytogenetic abnormality by itself should allow the diagnosis of MDS is a matter of debate, as stated above. From the authors' experience, the number of cases with an MDS-typical cytogenetic aberration without morphologic abnormalities (mostly del(20q)) is extremely rare, indeed. Also, the number of cases with dysplasia in the bone marrow without cytopenia, a condition dubbed idiopathic dysplasia of unknown significance is even rarer. Because morphology is not the Holy Grail, additional supportive investigations, including flow cytometry and molecular genetics, are direly needed to substantiate the diagnosis in difficult cases. Whether conventional morphology will finally end up in the history books may be possible, but seems unlikely at present.

DISCLOSURE

The authors declare no conflict of interest. This work has been supported by the German Kompetenznetz "akute und chronische Leukämien".

REFERENCES

1. Bain BJ. Dyserythropoiesis in visceral leishmaniasis. Am J Hematol 2010;85:781.
2. Dawson MA, Davis A, Elliott P, et al. Linezolid-induced dyserythropoiesis: chloramphenicol toxicity revisited. Intern Med J 2005;35:626–8.
3. Goasguen JE, Bennett JM, Bain BJ, et al. Dyserythropoiesis in the diagnosis of the myelodysplastic syndromes and other myeloid neoplasms: problem areas. Br J Haematol 2018;182:526–33.
4. Lu PL, Hsiao HH, Tsai JJ, et al. Dengue virus-associated hemophagocytic syndrome and dyserythropoiesis: a case report. Kaohsiung J Med Sci 2005;21:34–9.
5. Lv C, Xu Y, Wang J, et al. Dysplastic changes in erythroid precursors as a manifestation of lead poisoning: report of a case and review of literature. Int J Clin Exp Pathol 2015;8:818–23.
6. Siddiqui S, Ramlal R. "Myelodysplasia" from copper deficiency. Blood 2019; 133:883.
7. Wickramasinghe SN, Looareesuwan S, Nagachinta B, et al. Dyserythropoiesis and ineffective erythropoiesis in Plasmodium vivax malaria. Br J Haematol 1989;72:91–9.
8. Zanella A, Bianchi P, Fermo E. Pyruvate kinase deficiency. Haematologica 2007; 92:721–3.
9. Matsuda A, Kawabata H, Tohyama K, et al. Interobserver concordance of assessments of dysplasia and blast counts for the diagnosis of patients with cytopenia: from the Japanese central review study. Leuk Res 2018;74:137–43.
10. Malcovati L, Cazzola M. The shadowlands of MDS: idiopathic cytopenias of undetermined significance (ICUS) and clonal hematopoiesis of indeterminate potential (CHIP). Hematology Am Soc Hematol Educ Program 2015;2015:299–307.
11. Valent P, Orazi A, Steensma DP, et al. Proposed minimal diagnostic criteria for myelodysplastic syndromes (MDS) and potential pre-MDS conditions. Oncotarget 2017;8:73483–500.
12. Arber DA, Orazi A, Hasserjian R, et al. The 2016 revision to the World Health Organization classification of myeloid neoplasms and acute leukemia. Blood 2016; 127:2391–405.
13. Bejar R, Stevenson KE, Caughey B, et al. Somatic mutations predict poor outcome in patients with myelodysplastic syndrome after hematopoietic stem-cell transplantation. J Clin Oncol 2014;32:2691–8.
14. Steensma DP, Bejar R, Jaiswal S, et al. Clonal hematopoiesis of indeterminate potential and its distinction from myelodysplastic syndromes. Blood 2015;126:9–16.
15. Valent P, Kern W, Hoermann G, et al. Clonal hematopoiesis with oncogenic potential (CHOP): separation from CHIP and roads to AML. Int J Mol Sci 2019;20 [pii: E789].
16. Glenn TC. Field guide to next-generation DNA sequencers. Mol Ecol Resour 2011;11:759–69.
17. Fox EJ, Reid-Bayliss KS, Emond MJ, et al. Accuracy of next generation sequencing platforms. Next Gener Seq Appl 2014;1:1000106.
18. Bejar R. Myelodysplastic syndromes diagnosis: what is the role of molecular testing? Curr Hematol Malig Rep 2015;10:282–91.
19. Mufti GJ, Bennett JM, Goasguen J, et al. Diagnosis and classification of myelodysplastic syndrome: International Working Group on Morphology of myelodysplastic syndrome (IWGM-MDS) consensus proposals for the definition and enumeration of myeloblasts and ring sideroblasts. Haematologica 2008;93: 1712–7.

20. Berger R, Bernheim A, Daniel MT, et al. Cytologic characterization and significance of normal karyotypes in t(8;21) acute myeloblastic leukemia. Blood 1982;59:171–8.
21. Giagounidis AA, Hildebrandt B, Braunstein S, et al. Testicular infiltration in acute myeloid leukemia with complex karyotype including t(8;21). Ann Hematol 2002; 81:115–8.

Genetic Predisposition to Myelodysplastic Syndrome in Clinical Practice

Kristen E. Schratz, MD[a,b], Amy E. DeZern, MD, MHS[b,c],*

KEYWORDS

- Myelodysplastic syndrome • Inherited predisposition • Germline mutations
- Somatic mutations • Diagnostic testing • Hematopoietic stem cell transplant

KEY POINTS

- Inherited predisposition to myelodysplastic syndrome (MDS) and acute myeloid leukemia (AML) occurs in children as well as older adults.
- Analysis of the genetics of the disease is now standard of care in the evaluation of patients with MDS.
- Patients without syndromic features and negative family histories can still have a germline predisposition to MDS.
- Somatic tumor panels cannot replace dedicated genetic evaluations for germline mutations in the many genes implicated in genetic predisposition to MDS/AML.
- Diagnosis of an inherited predisposition has important implications for counseling and management.

INTRODUCTION

The myelodysplastic syndromes (MDS) are a heterogeneous group of clonal hematopoietic stem cell disorders that typically affect older adults (median age, 76 years[1]) but do occur less commonly in children and young adults. There is increasing recognition of an inherited predisposition to MDS as well as acute myeloid leukemia (AML) in both children and older individuals. Specific syndromes and gene mutations are infrequent but, collectively, inherited predisposition to myeloid malignancy represents a significant proportion of these diagnoses, with at least 5% of cases having a germline cause[2,3] and with a prevalence up to

[a] Division of Pediatric Oncology, Johns Hopkins University School of Medicine, Bloomberg 11379, 1800 Orleans Street, Baltimore, MD 21287, USA; [b] Sidney Kimmel Comprehensive Cancer Center, Johns Hopkins University School of Medicine, 1650 Orleans Street, Baltimore, MD 21287, USA; [c] Division of Hematologic Malignancies, Johns Hopkins University School of Medicine, CRBI Room 3M87, 1650 Orleans Street, Baltimore, MD 21287-0013, USA
* Corresponding author. Division of Hematologic Malignancies, Johns Hopkins University School of Medicine, CRBI Room 3M87, 1650 Orleans Street, Baltimore, MD 21287-0013.
E-mail address: adezern1@jhmi.edu

Hematol Oncol Clin N Am 34 (2020) 333–356
https://doi.org/10.1016/j.hoc.2019.10.002
0889-8588/20/© 2019 Elsevier Inc. All rights reserved.

10% to 15% in certain patient cohorts.[4–8] Germline predisposition to MDS can occur as a part of a syndrome or multisystem disorder or as a seemingly sporadic disease. The timely diagnosis of an underlying genetic predisposition is critical because it has broad implications for treatment, transplant considerations, long-term surveillance, and family counseling. It is more common for pediatric providers to consider these phenotypes, and thus increasing awareness for adult providers is becoming more important as clinicians realize that these disorders can present in older patients too. This article highlights the current state of knowledge for germline genetic causes of MDS (in children and adults); in addition, it provides a framework for the diagnosis and management of genetic predisposition to MDS/AML in the clinic for patients of all ages.

GERMLINE MYELODYSPLASTIC SYNDROME PREDISPOSITION SYNDROMES

Because of the increasing recognition of germline predisposition to MDS/AML and the impact on clinical care, germline predisposition to myeloid neoplasm was incorporated into the World Health Organization classification, and diagnostic recommendations were added to the most recent National Comprehensive Cancer Network (NCCN) practice guidelines.[9,10] NCCN guidelines provide relevant guidance on how to test patients but are lacking in explanations to clinicians for identification of appropriate candidates for testing. As such, some institutions have developed their own approach to the diagnosis and management of hereditary myeloid malignancies,[6,11–13] and consensus guidelines for surveillance and management exist for several specific MDS predisposition syndromes.[14–16] Common to all of these approaches is the appreciation that patients can have a germline predisposition to MDS with the absence of other syndromic features on history and physical and without a family history. Atypical or cryptic cases of the classic pediatric bone marrow failure (BMF) syndromes can become apparent only in adulthood, and MDS or AML can be the first presenting feature of these syndromes.

The major hereditary MDS/AML syndromes to date are summarized in **Table 1** with references to large case series detailing comprehensive features of each syndrome that have been published since the genetic diagnosis was established. The syndromes can be divided into the following categories:

1. Myeloid neoplasms with germline predisposition without a preexisting disorder or organ dysfunction (*CEBPA, DDX41*)
2. Myeloid neoplasms with germline predisposition and preexisting platelet disorders (*RUNX1, ANKRD26, ETV6*)
3. Myeloid neoplasms with germline predisposition and other organ dysfunction (*GATA2*, short telomere syndromes, other inherited BMF syndromes)
4. Traditional hereditary cancer predisposition syndromes (now understood to include hematologic malignancies in addition to solid tumors)

INDICATIONS FOR GENETIC TESTING

Certain clinical and laboratory features enrich for populations with inherited predisposition, and those populations warrant comprehensive screening for germline mutations as outlined later. However, limiting testing to only these high-risk patients could overlook a diagnosis in those older patients, nonsyndromic patients, or patients without family history who present with what seems to be de novo MDS but who carry a genetic predisposition.

Table 1
Genes involved in predisposition to myelodysplastic syndrome/acute myeloid leukemia and important clinical features

Syndrome	Gene(s)	Inheritance Mutation Types	Age of MDS/ AML Onset (range, y)	Hematologic Features	Extrahematopoietic Features	Other Cancers	Implications for Management	References
Myeloid Neoplasms with Germline Predisposition Without Preexisting Disorder or Organ Dysfunction
Familial AML with CEBPA mutations	CEBPA	AD Missense, FS	Adult>Ped (range 1–62)	AML	—	—	Chemosensitive Risk of second primary AML	47,48,81–86
Familial MDS/ AML with mutated DDX41	DDX41	AD Missense, FS, NS, CNV	Older adult (range 40–89)	MDS, AML, CML Lymphoma	Granulomatous and autoimmune disorders in a few families	—	—	70,87–91
Myeloid neoplasms with germline predisposition and preexisting platelet disorders
ANKRD26-related thrombo-cytopenia	ANKRD26	AD UTR variants; coding NS, missense[a]	Adult (range 26–70)	MDS, AML, CML CMML, CLL Thrombocytopenia	—	—	Mild bleeding tendency	92–98

(continued on next page)

Table 1
(continued)

Syndrome	Gene(s)	Inheritance Mutation Types	Age of MDS/ AML Onset (range, y)	Hematologic Features	Extrahematopoietic Features	Other Cancers	Implications for Management	References
ETV6-related thrombocytopenia	ETV6	AD Missense, FS, NS	Ped-Adult (range 8-82)	B-ALL, MDS, AML, CMML, DLBCL Variable thrombocytopenia	Not shared across pedigrees (developmental delay, dysmorphisms, autoimmunities)	Colon, breast, meningioma	Mild to moderate bleeding tendency	99-106
Familial platelet disorder with propensity to AML	RUNX1	AD Missense, FS, NS, CNV, rearrangements	Adult>Ped (range 5-72)	MDS, AML, T-ALL, hairy cell leukemia, CMML Mild to moderate thrombocytopenia	Case report of co-occurring eczema	—	—	50,112-120
Myeloid neoplasms with germline predisposition and other organ dysfunction								
Germline SAMD9/ SAMD9L	SAMD9 SAMD9L	AD Missense	Ped, rare adult (range 1-56)	AA, MDS, AML, CMML[a] Increased prevalence of monosomy 7	MIRAGE syndrome (SAMD9) Ataxia-Pancytopenia (SAMD9L)	—	—	7,37,38,121-124

Familial MDS/ AML with GATA2 mutation	GATA2	AD Missense, NS, FS, splicing, regulatory, CNV	AYA (range 3–78)	AA, MDS, AML, CMML Increased prevalence of monosomy 7	Infection Lymphedema Pulmonary alveolar proteinosis Hearing loss	—	8,19,44,65,107–111
Diamond-Blackfan anemia	GATA1 RPL5 RPL11 RPL15 RPL23 RPL26 RPL27 RPL31 RPL35a RPL36 RPS7 RPS10 RPS15 RPS17 RPS19 RPS24 RPS26 RPS27 RPS27A RPS28 RPS29 TSR2	AD, X linked (GATA1, TSR2) Missense, FS, NS, splicing, CNV, 3′ UTR	Adult>Ped (range 2–57)	Red cell aplasia, MDS, AML	Growth retardation, congenital malformations	Osteosarcoma, colon, possibly others	69,125–128

(continued on next page)

Table 1
(continued)

Syndrome	Gene(s)	Inheritance Mutation Types	Age of MDS/ AML Onset (range, y)	Hematologic Features	Extrahematopoietic Features	Other Cancers	Implications for Management	References
Fanconi anemia	FANCA FANCB FANCC FANCD1/BRCA2 FANCD2 FANCE FANCF FANCG FANCI FANCJ/BRIP1 FANCL FANCM FANCN/PALB2 FANCO/RAD51C FANCP/SLX4 FANCQ/ERCC4 FANCR/RAD51 FANCS/BRCA1 FANCT/UBE2T FANCU/XRCC2 FANCV	AR AD (FANCR) X linked (FANCB) Missense, FS, NS, splicing, CNV	AYA (range 1–57)	AA, MDS, AML ALL with FANCD1	Short stature, developmental delay, skeletal and renal abnormalities	SCC of head, neck and anogenital region	Require attenuated therapy, radiosensitive	61,69,129–132

Syndrome	Genes	Inheritance / Mutation type	Age (population)	Hematologic malignancy	Non-hematologic features	Other cancers	Treatment considerations	References
Short telomere syndromes	ACD/TPP1, CTC1, DKC1, NAF1, NHP2, NOP10, PARN, POT1, RTEL1, TR, TERT, TINF2, WRAP53/TCAB1, ZCCHC8	AD, AR, X linked Missense, FS, NS, splicing, CNV TR: SNV, INDELs	Adult>Ped (range 2–77)	AA, MDS, AML	Mucocutaneous features, pulmonary fibrosis, liver disease, immunodeficiency, enteropathy, severe congenital anomalies in some	SCC of head, neck and anogenital region	Attenuated regimen, radiosensitive	69,79,80,133–144
Shwachman-Diamond	SBDS, DNAJC21, EFL1	AR Missense, FS, NS, splicing, CNV	AYA (range 2–53)	Neutropenia, MDS, AML	Exocrine pancreatic insufficiency, neurodevelopmental and skeletal abnormalities	—	—	2,38,69,145–147
Traditional Hereditary Cancer Predisposition Syndromes								
Li-Fraumeni	TP53, CHEK2	AD Missense, FS, NS, splicing, intronic, CNV	Ped + adult (range 4–50)	ALL, MDS, AML, CML, lymphoma	—	Breast, sarcoma, CNS, adreno cortical carcinoma	—	6,148–152

Abbreviations: AA, aplastic anemia; AD, autosomal dominant; ALL, acute lymphoblastic leukemia; AR, autosomal recessive; AYA, adolescent and young adult population; CLL, chronic lymphocytic leukemia; CML, chronic myeloid leukemia; CMML, chronic myelomonocytic leukemia; CNV, copy number variant; DLBCL, diffuse large B-cell lymphoma; FS, frameshift; MIRAGE, myelodysplasia, infection, restriction of growth, adrenal hypoplasia, genital phenotypes and enteropathy; NS, nonsense; Ped, pediatric-onset disease; SCC, squamous cell carcinoma.

[a] Finding reported in a single family or case report.

Germline genetic testing is recommended in:

- Young-onset MDS, before 50 years of age; a proportion have negative family history and no other suggestive features
- MDS with any clinical or pathologic feature of a BMF syndrome (including lifelong history of cytopenias, even if MDS diagnosis made at a later age)
- Familial cases with MDS, acute leukemia, aplastic anemia, unexplained cytopenias, or bleeding history in 2 or more relatives (first or second degree)
- Individuals or families with MDS/AML clustering with extrahematopoietic manifestations characteristic of the BMF syndromes (see **Table 1**)
- Personal history of MDS and multiple primary malignancies and/or strong family history of cancers at early ages
- Individuals with mutations in genes known to be associated with hereditary MDS/AML found on somatic tumor testing (discussed later)

Consider germline genetic testing in:

- Hypoplastic MDS at any age (without paroxysmal nocturnal hemoglobinuria [PNH] clone)
- Personal history of thrombocytopenia (diagnosed as autoimmune) not responsive to standard therapies
- Patients with chemotherapy toxicity more severe than experienced by most patients
- Related donor with unexplained cytopenias or poor peripheral blood stem cell mobilization; donor-derived malignancy after related donor hematopoietic stem cell transplant (HSCT)
- Certain patients with therapy-related myeloid malignancies may be more likely to harbor germline variants in predisposition genes

EVALUATION FOR GERMLINE PREDISPOSITION TO MYELODYSPLASTIC SYNDROME

Standard diagnostic criteria for MDS apply to patients with germline predisposition and all the conventional diagnostic evaluations should be done. The underlying germline predisposition may not be evident on usual evaluations, so a high index of suspicion and dedicated work-up are needed. Mutations in some of the genes known to cause hereditary myeloid malignancy, such as *CEBPA*, *RUNX1*, or *TP53*, can also arise somatically in the clonal MDS/AML population. Clinically theses scenarios can lack clarity without further evaluation. Published guidelines now include consideration of additional molecular and genetic testing specifically for hereditary hematologic malignancies.[10] Patients should receive both pretest and posttest counseling according to standard genetic testing clinical practice guidelines.[17,18]

Bone Marrow Studies

MDS arising from an underlying marrow failure state can have distinguishing syndrome-specific features[19–21] or can appear to be sporadic MDS. A marrow evaluation is imperative in all cases. In the case of a hypocellular or patchy marrow in which MDS is suspected, increased cluster of differentiation (CD) 34 count, which can be quantified by flow cytometry of bone marrow aspirates or immunohistochemistry on the core biopsy, favors hypoplastic MDS rather than aplastic anemia.[22,23] Cytogenetics may also not grow or be nondiagnostic, and in that case fluorescence in situ hybridization (FISH) studies can be added to evaluate for the common aberrations.[13,24] In patients with noninformative or nondiagnostic cytogenetics, in cases in which this information may change management, single nucleotide polymorphism

(SNP) microarrays could be considered as an alternative karyotyping tool to detect most cytogenetic aberrations.[25–27] In patients with cytopenias and suspicion of an inherited syndrome, repeat marrow examinations may be necessary to establish the diagnosis of MDS because of hypocellular or patchy marrows and background dysplasia. This testing can be done at the time of clinical changes with the interval between marrows informed by the severity of cytopenias.

Tiered Approached to Genetic Testing

The authors' practice is to use a stepwise approach to the genetic evaluation of patients with MDS (**Fig. 1**). The tiered methodology allows for attention to detail, managing appropriate patient-centered issues, and parallel testing (of potential donor) if appropriate or necessary; there must also be acknowledgment of both the financial and emotional cost of these pathways at the bedside. In patients in whom there is a presumed higher risk for a genetic predisposition to MDS or features suspicious for these diagnoses, initial screening is done from the peripheral blood if applicable. Notably these tests include flow cytometry for a PNH clone,[28] especially if hypoplastic; telomere length measurement by CLIA (Clinical Laboratory Improvement Amendments)-certified flow cytometry and FISH (flowFISH)[29]; and chromosome breakage with diepoxybutane (DEB).[30] Polymerase chain reaction–based quantification of telomere length is not a reliable measure and should not be used in clinical settings.[29,31] The results of these initial tests help to further guide appropriate germline genetic testing.

The benefit of this approach is that these tests can be readily done from peripheral blood, are less expensive, and have a shorter turnaround time than most next-generation sequencing (NGS) platforms. This process quickly identifies patients at risk for short telomere syndromes and Fanconi anemia who are at high risk for increased toxicity from certain therapies, and the finding of a PNH clone, suggesting an acquired disorder, precludes the need for further genetic testing.[32] A tiered approach also allows for expectation management and reassurance to patients and families when possible. However, it can be less efficient, even if it is resource conscious. Further, it is important to facilitate appropriate work-up for both the patients and any related potential donors. Related donors should be screened in a targeted fashion if a predisposition syndrome is identified in the recipient. This screening is relevant for fully matched siblings or haploidentical siblings, children, or

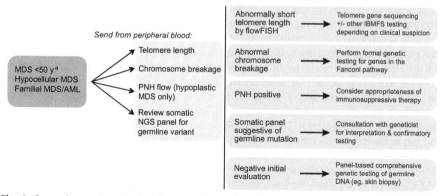

Fig. 1. Screening and evaluation for genetic predisposition to MDS. flowFISH, flow cytometry and FISH; IBMFS, inherited bone marrow failure syndrome; NGS, next-generation sequencing.
[a] Limiting screening to patients less than 50 years old misses cases of inherited MDS/AML.

parental donors. If the choice has been made a priori to use an unrelated donor, then the added stress of a familial work-up can be deferred or delayed until the patient has been treated.

Germline Source of DNA

It is critical at the bedside to evaluate the proper genetic material to document a germline disorder. Mutations in some of the genes known to cause hereditary myeloid malignancy can occur somatically. Thus, a germline source of DNA is imperative to distinguish acquired from inherited mutations. In addition, chromosomal aberrations and, in rare cases, revertant somatic mosaicism can obscure allele frequencies and may cause the genetic diagnosis to be missed if sequencing is only done from the peripheral blood.[33–38]

The preferred source of germline material for sequencing is DNA derived from skin fibroblasts cultured in a CLIA-certified laboratory.[39] Some sequencing laboratories require up to 5 μg of DNA for complete testing, which is difficult to obtain from other tissue sources (ie, hair roots and nail clippings[40]). Fibroblasts are usually obtained from a 3-mm skin punch biopsy, which can be done at the bedside even in very young patients or thrombocytopenic patients. Because of the time required to culture fibroblasts (3–6 weeks), a skin biopsy should be obtained as early as clinically feasible in the diagnostic evaluation. Saliva, buccal swab, and DNA from a skin biopsy directly yield sufficient DNA but can be contaminated with circulating cells.[41] In clinical situations in which a genetic diagnosis is needed urgently, these sources can be used initially with confirmatory testing done on cultured fibroblasts.[11]

Germline Next-Generation Sequencing Approaches

In the work-up of MDS, especially in adult hematology/oncology clinics, the use of NGS testing most often refers to targeted panels of somatic mutations known to be associated with myeloid malignancies.[42] These panels are distinct from alternative panels specific to germline mutations. Because of the phenotypic overlap of syndromes and nonclassic presentations, a comprehensive panel-based approach inclusive of the many genes implicated in genetic predisposition to MDS/AML is imperative.

Attention to the details of the testing ordered is vital because, without specific knowledge of the results obtained, false reassurance could come from a negative test that does not cover the relevant genetic markers for the inherited syndrome; this may require specific consultation with the genetic counselors as well as molecular pathologists before testing or at the time of interpretation of the results. The use of NGS methodology to detect point mutations in addition to copy number changes including large deletions/duplications is key.[4,43] It is also important that the NGS panel is specifically designed to capture certain noncoding regions that are known to be involved in disorders that predispose to MDS: the promoter in the 5′ untranslated region (UTR) of ANKRD26 (most families, reviewed by Godley[43]) and the enhancer region deep in intron 4 of GATA2 (NM_032638, accounting for at least 10% of families[8,44]). Capture of the UTR of ANRKD26 is variable on standard clinical whole-exome sequencing, and variants deep in the middle of the large GATA2 intron 4 are likely to be missed unless specifically targeted. Furthermore, somatic prognostic panels for MDS/AML, many of which include GATA2, do not capture these intronic variants nor report known pathogenic synonymous variants. There are several clinically available genetic testing panels for hereditary MDS/

AML, and testing methodology, genes included and interpretation expertise, in addition to turnaround time and cost, should be assessed prior to test selection.

Variants in Known Predisposition Genes Identified on Somatic Panels

As discussed earlier, it is recommended as standard of care to consider molecular testing for somatic mutations associated with MDS.[10] Increasingly these panels guide discussions of biology, prognosis, treatment pathways, and in rare instances targeted therapy on clinical trials. NGS of tumor samples using somatic panels may inadvertently identify patients at risk for germline predisposition to MDS/AML that were not otherwise appreciated to be high risk. Acquired pathogenic/likely pathogenic mutations in the same genes associated with genetic predisposition to MDS (*ANKRD26*, *CEBPA*, *DDX41*, *ETV6*, *GATA2*, *RUNX1*, or *TP53*) may be detected in more than 20% of patients tested with somatic myeloid malignancy panels.[45] Because of gross chromosomal rearrangements and more subtle gains and losses, the variant allele frequency of mutations in peripheral blood–derived DNA from patients with MDS is commonly unreliable, and deleterious variants identified on prognostic panels, especially in *DDX41* and *GATA2*,[45] should be investigated for germline origin regardless of allele frequency.[46] Ten percent of patients with biallelic *CEBPA* variants possess 1 of the 2 mutations in their germlines.[47,48] In genes such as *RUNX1* and *TP53*, the same variants can occur either in the germline or somatically in the MDS/AML clone. In these cases, the presence of a variant in the Catalogue Of Somatic Mutations In Cancer (COSMIC) database does not preclude it from being carried in the germline.[49,50] Variants in other pathways, such as telomerase and telomere maintenance genes, are rarely found in sequenced MDS/AML samples.[51] Germline confirmatory testing should be done in these cases to assess whether the somatically detected variant is really in the germline. In contrast, it is noteworthy that the absence of pathogenic variants on somatic panels does not exclude a germline predisposition and should not be used as a substitute for dedicated germline testing.

Interpretation of Somatic Gene Variants with Germline Allele Frequencies

In general, variants with allele frequencies between 40% and 60% could be germline, as opposed to acquired, in the malignant population. When these occur in genes known to be associated with an MDS predisposition syndrome, as described earlier and in **Table 1**, further consideration is warranted. When the variant occurs in genes known only to have a somatic role in MDS/AML, the clinician should be cautious before ascribing too much significance to it. It is possible that the variant could still be somatic and the allele frequency explained by the disease burden at the time of testing, or it could be a germline benign polymorphism. These potentially germline and inheritable variants should be approached carefully so as to ensure proper counseling but also avoidance of undue testing burden.

Interpretation of Germline Variants of Unknown Significance

When reviewing the results of somatic panel testing, it is possible for mutations that have a germline association to receive annotation. How these are codified and interpreted may vary by report. Interpretation of dedicated germline sequencing should be done according to guidelines for variant classification from the American College of Medical Genetics and Genomics, which recommends identified variants be assigned 1 of 5 categories: pathogenic, likely pathogenic, uncertain significance, likely benign, and benign.[52] In patients referred to the laboratory in an academic center for panel-based testing of hereditary MDS/AML, a pathogenic or likely pathogenic variant established the diagnosis in 15-20% of patients, but more than one-third of the patients carried variants of uncertain significance (VUSs) in known genes.[4] VUSs pose a challenge to clinicians and patients; thus, consultation with a geneticist may be indicated. Extreme caution must be taken when basing treatment decisions on the presence of a VUS so as to avoid ascribing a disorder to a nonpathogenic mutation. All individuals carry numerous heterozygous nonsynonymous coding variants in their germlines, many of which are common in the general population and likely benign polymorphisms.[53] Determining the frequency of germline VUSs in the general population is useful in assessing their potential pathogenicity.[54] In a rare mendelian disorder such as these myeloid diseases and syndromes, an allele frequency in the general population that is greater than expected for the disorder is less likely to be driving the disease. However, this assumption is less reliable in diseases with later onset in life.[52,55,56] Functional studies, such as telomere length measurement or chromosome breakage, if not previously done, can aid in assessing the pathogenicity of VUSs where applicable. Use of genomic tumor boards or multidisciplinary groups with germline expertise, in practice at some institutions to assess VUSs, can aid in variant interpretation before clinical decisions are made.[57] Variant pathogenicity should also be reevaluated as new cohorts are sequenced and new evidence is accrued. For example, TERT variants A202T, H412Y, and A1046T were at one time thought to be pathogenic, but evidence now suggests these are common polymorphisms.[6,58,59] Additional assessments of variants, such as segregation of VUSs in asymptomatic relatives and in vitro functional studies, should be done on a research basis.

CLONAL HEMATOPOIESIS IN GERMLINE MYELODYSPLASTIC SYNDROMES

The mechanisms by which these germline predisposition syndromes are leukemogenic are not fully understood. There are a few recurrent chromosomal aberrations and somatic mutations that are important to highlight. These mutations can be seen recurrently within MDS/AML arising from a single syndrome, such as somatic TP53 mutations in Shwachman-Diamond, or shared across MDS arising from different syndromes, such as monosomy 7.

Recurrent Chromosomal Aberrations

The selective pressure of the failing marrow in several of the inherited BMF syndromes drives recurrent, nonrandom chromosomal aberrations,[13,24] which are not necessarily leukemogenic but can affect prognosis. There is an increased prevalence of monosomy 7 in genetically mediated MDS compared with de novo, most commonly reported to date in SAMD9/9L in younger children and GATA2 in adolescents, but this can also be seen in the other syndromes. The loss of chromosome 7 or del(7q) in patients with SAMD9/9L mutations (located on chromosome 7q) deletes the mutant allele, alleviating the growth repression caused by the gain-of-function germline mutation. The outcome of this acquired monosomy 7 ranges from normalization of the karyotype and bone marrow (through duplication of the nonmutated allele) or progression to advanced MDS, thought to occur through acquisition of additional somatic driver mutations. The functional role of monosomy 7 in GATA2-deficient BMF is less clear. Isochromosome 7q and del20q occur in Shwachman-Diamond syndrome,[60] and 1q+ and 3q26q29 amplifications are common in Fanconi anemia.[61–63] Recurrent changes may be found in other inherited BMF syndromes as more cases are systematically studied. Review of the literature, even for case reports at the time of identification of these changes in a single patient, will be important as additional knowledge emerges.

Clonal Evolution Through Acquired Mutations

Driver and cooperating mutations are important for the pathogenesis of both de novo MDS/AML and MDS arising from a germline predisposition. The understanding of these co-mutational patterns is rapidly evolving; these acquired mutations may explain some of the variable penetrance and expressivity seen within families. For this reason, it is vital in older patients with previously undiagnosed predisposition syndromes to have both somatic and germline testing if applicable. In addition, patients with therapy-related myeloid malignancies may be more likely to harbor germline variants in predisposition genes and should be considered for testing as well.[64]

In unaffected *RUNX1* carriers <50 years, 6 of 9 (67%) harbored detectable somatic mutations, and all of the patients with *RUNX1*-mediated MDS/AML (5 of 5) had somatic mutations, suggesting clonal hematopoiesis occurs before the development of overt MDS/AML in *RUNX1* carriers.[65] However, most of these mutations detected by exome sequencing occurred in genes different than those seen recurrently mutated in MDS. In patients with germline *GATA2* mutations who developed MDS/AML, three-quarters (22 of 29) harbored MDS-associated somatic mutations; recurrent mutations in *ASXL1* (40%, loss of function) and *STAG2* (28%) were most common.[66,67] In relatives also carrying *GATA2* mutations but without MDS, it was less common for those with essentially normal marrows to have somatic driver mutations (1 of 5 studied), whereas, in those with abnormal marrows, 5 of 7 had somatic mutations, including 3 with *ASXL1*, suggesting this may be an intermediate phenotype in transition to an MDS state.[67]

Acquired *TP53* mutations were seen in 7 of 7 young adults with biallelic SBDS mutations before HSCT for MDS.[2] Further, ultradeep sequencing of patients with Shwachman-Diamond without MDS/AML has also identified acquired *TP53* mutations in half (13 of 27 patients), although at exceptionally low allele frequencies (median 0.36%, range 0.05%–3.1%) of unclear clinical significance.[68] The role of these recurrent events in the transformation to MDS/AML is an active area of research. Application of these somatic findings to monitoring and prevention is not yet established. Furthermore, the lack of prospective observational data limits the clinical ability to incorporate the knowledge of somatic variants' presence for prognostication in predisposed patients before the development of MDS.

SURVEILLANCE AND MANAGEMENT

There are many bedside benefits of real-time diagnosis of a germline MDS predisposition disorder. Some germline MDS predisposition disorders are characterized by extrahematopoietic manifestations, which can contribute to significant morbidity and for which screening can change management (see **Table 1**). Another important clinical advantage is insight into the natural history of the disorder. Most importantly, the added knowledge of a germline syndrome can alter or facilitate more appropriate therapy in affected individuals. Presumed lack of responsiveness to noncurative therapies for a germline disease likely prompts HSCT evaluation sooner from an unrelated donor. Recognition of the possibility of these diagnostic and treatment interactions is only the first step and then appropriate referrals with the use of resources can follow.[71]

Selection of Related Donors

Recognition of an inherited disorder is important before assessment and selection of a related donor. Unexplained cytopenias, recurrent/severe infections, or failure to mobilize stem cells in a donor may be caused by an underlying marrow failure syndrome and warrant additional investigation. However, completely asymptomatic related donors may still be carriers of the familial mutation because there can be significant heterogeneity for hematologic and extrahematopoietic manifestations within and across families carrying the same mutation. If a mutation has been identified in the recipient, potential related donors should be counseled and then offered targeted testing to screen for this mutation. Results of this testing are important both for decision on use as a donor as well as to identify the person's own potential predisposition and disease risk. These aspects should be explained clearly to the patient and related donor as the process is ongoing. Using a related donor carrying the familial mutation puts both the donor and recipient at risk for complication.[72,73]

If the personal or family history is suspicious for a germline MDS predisposition syndrome but no causative mutation can be identified, an attempt should be made to find a matched unrelated donor in hopes of avoidance of the conceivable risk of transplanting the causative mutation. If there is no HLA-matched unrelated donor or there is an urgent indication for HSCT, the potential risks and benefits should be discussed with both the recipient and the donor.[73] It is also possible to use second-degree relatives as haploidentical donors, so there may be less traditional options to find a suitable donor for potentially curative HSCT in these families as well.[74] Regardless, bone marrow studies and thorough hematologic evaluation in relatives under consideration for allograft donation is strongly encouraged.

Recipient Specific Implications

Diagnosis of a germline MDS predisposition disorder also has implications for timing of transplant, preparative regimens, and posttransplant care. Understanding the natural history of individual disorders is critical to making decisions at the bedside. Patients with Fanconi anemia and short telomere syndromes can experience increased toxicity from standard chemotherapy and radiation and need attenuated regimens; however, there is more published experience with HSCT for BMF than MDS.[75–77] Patients with short telomere syndromes post-HSCT continue to be at risk for additional short telomere manifestations as they age, which can occur at an earlier age in this setting. Patients with Fanconi anemia have an increased cancer risk post-HSCT.[69,78] Patients with germline CEBPA mutations are at risk of second primary AMLs, but prospective trials have not been done to assess the best timing for HSCT in this situation.

Familial Implications

Identification of a genetic predisposition to MDS has implications for both the immediate and extended family. This possibility should be discussed with the patients by genetic counselors or clinicians experienced in these issues before genetic testing is pursued. In children, parental testing to determine whether a variant is inherited or de novo should be obtained before screening asymptomatic siblings. Genetic testing of asymptomatic individuals, especially children, should only be undertaken after consultation of risks and benefits with a genetic counselor. This consultation can become more complicated with adult children of older patients with MDS, given that it is less expected in these ages to diagnose a germline condition. Dialogues surrounding the repercussions must be had transparently with all those involved.

EMERGING IDEAS
Discovery

The genetic cause for more than half of familial MDS/AML cases remains unsolved.[6,38,65,80] Further study of these families, especially of those who present as adults, has the potential to identify new mechanisms of disease in known genes (regulatory mutations, synonymous mutations) and identify new genes and pathways. This knowledge will aid in diagnosis, surveillance, and management, and also may provide insight into leukemogenic mechanisms for prevention and targeted therapy in both germline and somatic conditions.

Prevention and Treatment

Increasing use of targeted treatments in MDS/AML may apply to familial cases with sporadic mutations in these same pathways. Understanding of the pathogenesis in specific syndromes may also lead to targeted therapies that can be used for prevention of MDS/AML. It is hoped that additional investigation of genetic and epigenetic alterations in these patients will elucidate the mechanisms of reduced penetrance in some syndromes and also lead to prevention strategies. Acquisition of multiple somatic mutations in genes recurrently mutated in myeloid malignancy is high risk for transformation. No prospective trials exist to guide treatment decisions, but consideration of intervention should be discussed with the patient.

SUMMARY

Germline predisposition to MDS, even in adults, is more common than was previously recognized and important to diagnose in real time before treatment, and especially before HSCT. Individual syndromes may be rare but, collectively, represent a significant risk in both pediatric and adult patients. Awareness of the risk as well as methods of identification are increasingly important steps in providing high-quality care to all patients with MDS. Growing knowledge about this has the potential to lead to personalized treatment paradigms for these patients that also have broader implications for the more numerous patients with somatic mutations in similar pathways.

ACKNOWLEDGEMENTS

The work of K.E.S. is supported by NIH T32HL007525.

DISCLOSURE

The authors declare no relevant conflicts of interest.

REFERENCES

1. Ma X. Epidemiology of myelodysplastic syndromes. Am J Med 2012;125(7 Suppl):S2–5.
2. Lindsley RC, Saber W, Mar BG, et al. Prognostic mutations in myelodysplastic syndrome after stem-cell transplantation. N Engl J Med 2017;376(6):536–47.
3. Zhang J, Nichols KE, Downing JR. Germline mutations in predisposition genes in pediatric cancer. N Engl J Med 2016;374(14):1391.
4. Guidugli L, Johnson AK, Alkorta-Aranburu G, et al. Clinical utility of gene panel-based testing for hereditary myelodysplastic syndrome/acute leukemia predisposition syndromes. Leukemia 2017;31(5):1226–9.
5. Hirsch CM, Przychodzen BP, Radivoyevitch T, et al. Molecular features of early onset adult myelodysplastic syndrome. Haematologica 2017;102(6):1028–34.
6. Keel SB, Scott A, Sanchez-Bonilla M, et al. Genetic features of myelodysplastic syndrome and aplastic anemia in pediatric and young adult patients. Haematologica 2016;101(11):1343–50.
7. Schwartz JR, Ma J, Lamprecht T, et al. The genomic landscape of pediatric myelodysplastic syndromes. Nat Commun 2017;8(1):1557.

8. Wlodarski MW, Hirabayashi S, Pastor V, et al. Prevalence, clinical characteristics, and prognosis of GATA2-related myelodysplastic syndromes in children and adolescents. Blood 2016;127(11):1387–97 [quiz: 1518].

9. Arber DA, Orazi A, Hasserjian R, et al. The 2016 revision to the World Health Organization classification of myeloid neoplasms and acute leukemia. Blood 2016; 127(20):2391–405.

10. Greenberg PL, Stone RM, Al-Kali A, et al. Myelodysplastic syndromes, version 2.2017, NCCN clinical practice guidelines in oncology. J Natl Compr Canc Netw 2017;15(1):60–87.

11. University of Chicago Hematopoietic Malignancies Cancer Risk Team. How I diagnose and manage individuals at risk for inherited myeloid malignancies. Blood 2016;128(14):1800–13.

12. DiNardo CD, Bannon SA, Routbort M, et al. Evaluation of patients and families with concern for predispositions to hematologic malignances within the hereditary Hematologic Malignancy Clinic (HHMC). Clin Lymphoma Myeloma Leuk 2016;16(7):417–28.e2.

13. Godley LA, Shimamura A. Genetic predisposition to hematologic malignancies: management and surveillance. Blood 2017;130(4):424–32.

14. Frohnmayer D, Frohnmayer L, Guinan E, et al. Fanconi Anemia: Guidelines for Diagnosis and Management. 4th edition. Eugene, (OR): Fanconi Anemia Research Fund, Inc; 2014.

15. Vlachos A, Ball S, Dahl N, et al. Diagnosing and treating Diamond Blackfan anaemia: results of an international clinical consensus conference. Br J Haematol 2008;142(6):859–76.

16. Savage SA, Cook EF. Dyskeratosis Congenita and Telomere Biology Disorders: Diagnosis and Management Guidelines. 1st edition. New York: Dyskeratosis Congenita Outreach, Inc; 2015.

17. Lu KH, Wood ME, Daniels M, et al. American Society of Clinical Oncology Expert Statement: collection and use of a cancer family history for oncology providers. J Clin Oncol 2014;32(8):833–40.

18. Stanislaw C, Xue Y, Wilcox WR. Genetic evaluation and testing for hereditary forms of cancer in the era of next-generation sequencing. Cancer Biol Med 2016;13(1):55–67.

19. Calvo KR, Vinh DC, Maric I, et al. Myelodysplasia in autosomal dominant and sporadic monocytopenia immunodeficiency syndrome: diagnostic features and clinical implications. Haematologica 2011;96(8):1221–5.

20. Proytcheva MA. Diagnostic pediatric hematopathology. Cambridge (United Kingdom): Cambridge University Press; 2011.

21. Kallen ME, Dulau-Florea A, Wang W, et al. Acquired and germline predisposition to bone marrow failure: Diagnostic features and clinical implications. Semin Hematol 2019;56(1):69–82.

22. Matsui WH, Brodsky RA, Smith BD, et al. Quantitative analysis of bone marrow CD34 cells in aplastic anemia and hypoplastic myelodysplastic syndromes. Leukemia 2006;20(3):458–62.

23. DeZern AE, Sekeres MA. The challenging world of cytopenias: distinguishing myelodysplastic syndromes from other disorders of marrow failure. Oncologist 2014;19(7):735–45.

24. Kennedy AL, Shimamura A. Genetic predisposition to MDS: clinical features and clonal evolution. Blood 2019;133(10):1071–85.

25. Medeiros BC, Othus M, Estey EH, et al. Unsuccessful diagnostic cytogenetic analysis is a poor prognostic feature in acute myeloid leukaemia. Br J Haematol 2014;164(2):245–50.

26. Tiu RV, Gondek LP, O'Keefe CL, et al. New lesions detected by single nucleotide polymorphism array-based chromosomal analysis have important clinical impact in acute myeloid leukemia. J Clin Oncol 2009;27(31):5219–26.

27. Dougherty MJ, Wilmoth DM, Tooke LS, et al. Implementation of high resolution single nucleotide polymorphism array analysis as a clinical test for patients with hematologic malignancies. Cancer Genet 2011;204(1):26–38.

28. Dezern AE, Borowitz MJ. ICCS/ESCCA consensus guidelines to detect GPI-deficient cells in paroxysmal nocturnal hemoglobinuria (PNH) and related disorders part 1 - clinical utility. Cytometry B Clin Cytom 2018;94(1):16–22.

29. Alder JK, Hanumanthu VS, Strong MA, et al. Diagnostic utility of telomere length testing in a hospital-based setting. Proc Natl Acad Sci U S A 2018;115(10): E2358–65.

30. Auerbach AD. Diagnosis of Fanconi anemia by diepoxybutane analysis. Curr Protoc Hum Genet 2015;85:8.7.1–17.

31. Martin-Ruiz CM, Baird D, Roger L, et al. Reproducibility of telomere length assessment–an international collaborative study. Int J Epidemiol 2015;44(5): 1749–54.

32. DeZern AE, Symons HJ, Resar LS, et al. Detection of paroxysmal nocturnal hemoglobinuria clones to exclude inherited bone marrow failure syndromes. Eur J Haematol 2014;92(6):467–70.

33. Alder JK, Stanley SE, Wagner CL, et al. Exome sequencing identifies mutant TINF2 in a family with pulmonary fibrosis. Chest 2015;147(5):1361–8.

34. Gross M, Hanenberg H, Lobitz S, et al. Reverse mosaicism in Fanconi anemia: natural gene therapy via molecular self-correction. Cytogenet Genome Res 2002;98(2–3):126–35.

35. Jongmans MC, Verwiel ET, Heijdra Y, et al. Revertant somatic mosaicism by mitotic recombination in dyskeratosis congenita. Am J Hum Genet 2012;90(3): 426–33.

36. Pastor VB, Sahoo SS, Boklan J, et al. Constitutional SAMD9L mutations cause familial myelodysplastic syndrome and transient monosomy 7. Haematologica 2018;103(3):427–37.

37. Tesi B, Davidsson J, Voss M, et al. Gain-of-function SAMD9L mutations cause a syndrome of cytopenia, immunodeficiency, MDS, and neurological symptoms. Blood 2017;129(16):2266–79.

38. Bluteau O, Sebert M, Leblanc T, et al. A landscape of germ line mutations in a cohort of inherited bone marrow failure patients. Blood 2018;131(7):717–32.

39. Teer JK, Zhang Y, Chen L, et al. Evaluating somatic tumor mutation detection without matched normal samples. Hum Genomics 2017;11(1):22.

40. Padron E, Ball MC, Teer JK, et al. Germ line tissues for optimal detection of somatic variants in myelodysplastic syndromes. Blood 2018;131(21):2402–5.

41. Looi ML, Zakaria H, Osman J, et al. Quantity and quality assessment of DNA extracted from saliva and blood. Clin Lab 2012;58(3–4):307–12.

42. Steensma DP. How I use molecular genetic tests to evaluate patients who have or may have myelodysplastic syndromes. Blood 2018;132(16):1657–63.

43. Godley LA. Inherited predisposition to acute myeloid leukemia. Semin Hematol 2014;51(4):306–21.

44. Hsu AP, Johnson KD, Falcone EL, et al. GATA2 haploinsufficiency caused by mutations in a conserved intronic element leads to MonoMAC syndrome. Blood 2013;121(19):3830–7. S3831-3837.

45. Drazer MW, Kadri S, Sukhanova M, et al. Prognostic tumor sequencing panels frequently identify germ line variants associated with hereditary hematopoietic malignancies. Blood Adv 2018;2(2):146–50.

46. Churpek JE. Familial myelodysplastic syndrome/acute myeloid leukemia. Best Pract Res Clin Haematol 2017;30(4):287–9.

47. Pabst T, Eyholzer M, Haefliger S, et al. Somatic CEBPA mutations are a frequent second event in families with germline CEBPA mutations and familial acute myeloid leukemia. J Clin Oncol 2008;26(31):5088–93.

48. Taskesen E, Bullinger L, Corbacioglu A, et al. Prognostic impact, concurrent genetic mutations, and gene expression features of AML with CEBPA mutations in a cohort of 1182 cytogenetically normal AML patients: further evidence for CEBPA double mutant AML as a distinctive disease entity. Blood 2011;117(8): 2469–75.

49. Osato M. Point mutations in the RUNX1/AML1 gene: another actor in RUNX leukemia. Oncogene 2004;23(24):4284–96.

50. Preudhomme C, Renneville A, Bourdon V, et al. High frequency of RUNX1 biallelic alteration in acute myeloid leukemia secondary to familial platelet disorder. Blood 2009;113(22):5583–7.

51. Walter MJ, Shen D, Shao J, et al. Clonal diversity of recurrently mutated genes in myelodysplastic syndromes. Leukemia 2013;27(6):1275–82.

52. Richards S, Aziz N, Bale S, et al. Standards and guidelines for the interpretation of sequence variants: a joint consensus recommendation of the American College of Medical Genetics and Genomics and the Association for Molecular Pathology. Genet Med 2015;17(5):405–24.

53. 1000 Genomes Project Consortium, Abecasis GR, Auton A, Brooks LD, et al. An integrated map of genetic variation from 1,092 human genomes. Nature 2012; 491(7422):56–65.

54. Karczewski K, Francioli LC, Tiao G, et al. Variation across 141,456 human exomes and genomes reveals the spectrum of loss-of-function intolerance across human protein-coding genes. bioRxiv 2019.

55. de Andrade KC, Frone MN, Wegman-Ostrosky T, et al. Variable population prevalence estimates of germline TP53 variants: a gnomAD-based analysis. Hum Mutat 2019;40(1):97–105.

56. Soussi T, Leroy B, Devir M, et al. High prevalence of cancer-associated TP53 variants in the gnomAD database: a word of caution concerning the use of variant filtering. Hum Mutat 2019;40(5):516–24.

57. van der Velden DL, van Herpen CML, van Laarhoven HWM, et al. Molecular Tumor Boards: current practice and future needs. Ann Oncol 2017;28(12):3070–5.

58. Alder JK, Chen JJ, Lancaster L, et al. Short telomeres are a risk factor for idiopathic pulmonary fibrosis. Proc Natl Acad Sci U S A 2008;105(35):13051–6.

59. Du HY, Pumbo E, Ivanovich J, et al. TERC and TERT gene mutations in patients with bone marrow failure and the significance of telomere length measurements. Blood 2009;113(2):309–16.

60. Maserati E, Minelli A, Pressato B, et al. Shwachman syndrome as mutator phenotype responsible for myeloid dysplasia/neoplasia through karyotype instability and chromosomes 7 and 20 anomalies. Genes Chromosomes Cancer 2006;45(4):375–82.

61. Cioc AM, Wagner JE, MacMillan ML, et al. Diagnosis of myelodysplastic syndrome among a cohort of 119 patients with fanconi anemia: morphologic and cytogenetic characteristics. Am J Clin Pathol 2010;133(1):92–100.

62. Quentin S, Cuccuini W, Ceccaldi R, et al. Myelodysplasia and leukemia of Fanconi anemia are associated with a specific pattern of genomic abnormalities that includes cryptic RUNX1/AML1 lesions. Blood 2011;117(15):e161–70.

63. Tonnies H, Huber S, Kuhl JS, et al. Clonal chromosomal aberrations in bone marrow cells of Fanconi anemia patients: gains of the chromosomal segment 3q26q29 as an adverse risk factor. Blood 2003;101(10):3872–4.

64. Churpek JE, Larson RA. The evolving challenge of therapy-related myeloid neoplasms. Best Pract Res Clin Haematol 2013;26(4):309–17.

65. Churpek JE, Pyrtel K, Kanchi KL, et al. Genomic analysis of germ line and somatic variants in familial myelodysplasia/acute myeloid leukemia. Blood 2015; 126(22):2484–90.

66. Ding LW, Ikezoe T, Tan KT, et al. Mutational profiling of a MonoMAC syndrome family with GATA2 deficiency. Leukemia 2017;31(1):244–5.

67. McReynolds LJ, Yang Y, Yuen Wong H, et al. MDS-associated mutations in germline GATA2 mutated patients with hematologic manifestations. Leuk Res 2019;76:70–5.

68. Xia J, Miller CA, Baty J, et al. Somatic mutations and clonal hematopoiesis in congenital neutropenia. Blood 2018;131(4):408–16.

69. Alter BP, Giri N, Savage SA, et al. Cancer in the National Cancer Institute inherited bone marrow failure syndrome cohort after fifteen years of follow-up. Haematologica 2018;103(1):30–9.

70. Quesada AE, Routbort MJ, DiNardo CD, et al. DDX41 mutations in myeloid neoplasms are associated with male gender, TP53 mutations and high-risk disease. Am J Hematol 2019;94(7):757–66.

71. Clifford M, Bannon S, Bednar EM, et al. Clinical applicability of proposed algorithm for identifying individuals at risk for hereditary hematologic malignancies. Leuk Lymphoma 2019;60(12):1–8.

72. Churpek JE, Artz A, Bishop M, et al. Correspondence regarding the consensus statement from the worldwide network for blood and marrow transplantation standing committee on donor issues. Biol Blood Marrow Transplant 2016; 22(1):183–4.

73. Gadalla SM, Wang T, Haagenson M, et al. Association between donor leukocyte telomere length and survival after unrelated allogeneic hematopoietic cell transplantation for severe aplastic anemia. JAMA 2015;313(6):594–602.

74. Elmariah H, Kasamon YL, Zahurak M, et al. Haploidentical bone marrow transplantation with post-transplant cyclophosphamide using non-first-degree related donors. Biol Blood Marrow Transplant 2018;24(5):1099–102.

75. Gadalla SM, Sales-Bonfim C, Carreras J, et al. Outcomes of allogeneic hematopoietic cell transplantation in patients with dyskeratosis congenita. Biol Blood Marrow Transplant 2013;19(8):1238–43.

76. Barbaro P, Vedi A. Survival after hematopoietic stem cell transplant in patients with dyskeratosis congenita: systematic review of the literature. Biol Blood Marrow Transplant 2016;22(7):1152–8.

77. Dietz AC, Orchard PJ, Baker KS, et al. Disease-specific hematopoietic cell transplantation: nonmyeloablative conditioning regimen for dyskeratosis congenita. Bone Marrow Transpl 2011;46(1):98–104.

78. Anur P, Friedman DN, Sklar C, et al. Late effects in patients with Fanconi anemia following allogeneic hematopoietic stem cell transplantation from alternative donors. Bone Marrow Transplant 2016;51(7):938–44.

79. Gable DL, Gaysinskaya V, Atik CC, et al. ZCCHC8, the nuclear exosome targeting component, is mutated in familial pulmonary fibrosis and is required for telomerase RNA maturation. Genes Dev 2019;33(19-20):1381–96.

80. Holme H, Hossain U, Kirwan M, et al. Marked genetic heterogeneity in familial myelodysplasia/acute myeloid leukaemia. Br J Haematol 2012;158(2):242–8.

81. Smith ML, Cavenagh JD, Lister TA, et al. Mutation of CEBPA in familial acute myeloid leukemia. N Engl J Med 2004;351(23):2403–7.

82. Sellick GS, Spendlove HE, Catovsky D, et al. Further evidence that germline CEBPA mutations cause dominant inheritance of acute myeloid leukaemia. Leukemia 2005;19(7):1276–8.

83. Stelljes M, Corbacioglu A, Schlenk RF, et al. Allogeneic stem cell transplant to eliminate germline mutations in the gene for CCAAT-enhancer-binding protein alpha from hematopoietic cells in a family with AML. Leukemia 2011;25(7): 1209–10.

84. Tawana K, Wang J, Renneville A, et al. Disease evolution and outcomes in familial AML with germline CEBPA mutations. Blood 2015;126(10):1214–23.

85. Pathak A, Seipel K, Pemov A, et al. Whole exome sequencing reveals a C-terminal germline variant in CEBPA-associated acute myeloid leukemia: 45-year follow up of a large family. Haematologica 2016;101(7):846–52.

86. Yan B, Ng C, Moshi G, et al. Myelodysplastic features in a patient with germline CEBPA-mutant acute myeloid leukaemia. J Clin Pathol 2016;69(7):652–4.

87. Polprasert C, Schulze I, Sekeres MA, et al. Inherited and somatic defects in DDX41 in myeloid neoplasms. Cancer cell 2015;27(5):658–70.

88. Cardoso SR, Ryan G, Walne AJ, et al. Germline heterozygous DDX41 variants in a subset of familial myelodysplasia and acute myeloid leukemia. Leukemia 2016;30(10):2083–6.

89. Lewinsohn M, Brown AL, Weinel LM, et al. Novel germ line DDX41 mutations define families with a lower age of MDS/AML onset and lymphoid malignancies. Blood 2016;127(8):1017–23.

90. Li R, Sobreira N, Witmer PD, et al. Two novel germline DDX41 mutations in a family with inherited myelodysplasia/acute myeloid leukemia. Haematologica 2016;101(6):e228–31.

91. Kobayashi S, Kobayashi A, Osawa Y, et al. Donor cell leukemia arising from pre-leukemic clones with a novel germline DDX41 mutation after allogenic hematopoietic stem cell transplantation. Leukemia 2017;31(4):1020–2.

92. Noris P, Perrotta S, Seri M, et al. Mutations in ANKRD26 are responsible for a frequent form of inherited thrombocytopenia: analysis of 78 patients from 21 families. Blood 2011;117(24):6673–80.

93. Pippucci T, Savoia A, Perrotta S, et al. Mutations in the 5' UTR of ANKRD26, the ankirin repeat domain 26 gene, cause an autosomal-dominant form of inherited thrombocytopenia, THC2. Am J Hum Genet 2011;88(1):115–20.

94. Al Daama SA, Housawi YH, Dridi W, et al. A missense mutation in ANKRD26 segregates with thrombocytopenia. Blood 2013;122(3):461–2.

95. Noris P, Favier R, Alessi MC, et al. ANKRD26-related thrombocytopenia and myeloid malignancies. Blood 2013;122(11):1987–9.

96. Marquez R, Hantel A, Lorenz R, et al. A new family with a germline ANKRD26 mutation and predisposition to myeloid malignancies. Leuk Lymphoma 2014; 55(12):2945–6.

97. Perez Botero J, Oliveira JL, Chen D, et al. ASXL1 mutated chronic myelomonocytic leukemia in a patient with familial thrombocytopenia secondary to germline mutation in ANKRD26. Blood Cancer J 2015;5:e315.

98. Marconi C, Canobbio I, Bozzi V, et al. 5'UTR point substitutions and N-terminal truncating mutations of ANKRD26 in acute myeloid leukemia. J Hematol Oncol 2017;10(1):18.

99. Moriyama T, Metzger ML, Wu G, et al. Germline genetic variation in ETV6 and risk of childhood acute lymphoblastic leukaemia: a systematic genetic study. Lancet Oncol 2015;16(16):1659–66.

100. Noetzli L, Lo RW, Lee-Sherick AB, et al. Germline mutations in ETV6 are associated with thrombocytopenia, red cell macrocytosis and predisposition to lymphoblastic leukemia. Nat Genet 2015;47(5):535–8.

101. Topka S, Vijai J, Walsh MF, et al. Germline ETV6 mutations confer susceptibility to acute lymphoblastic leukemia and thrombocytopenia. Plos Genet 2015;11(6): e1005262.

102. Zhang MY, Churpek JE, Keel SB, et al. Germline ETV6 mutations in familial thrombocytopenia and hematologic malignancy. Nat Genet 2015;47(2):180–5.

103. Melazzini F, Palombo F, Balduini A, et al. Clinical and pathogenic features of ETV6-related thrombocytopenia with predisposition to acute lymphoblastic leukemia. Haematologica 2016;101(11):1333–42.

104. Poggi M, Canault M, Favier M, et al. Germline variants in ETV6 underlie reduced platelet formation, platelet dysfunction and increased levels of circulating CD34+ progenitors. Haematologica 2017;102(2):282–94.

105. Di Paola J, Porter CC. ETV6-related thrombocytopenia and leukemia predisposition. Blood 2019;134(8):663–7.

106. Rampersaud E, Ziegler DS, Iacobucci I, et al. Germline deletion of ETV6 in familial acute lymphoblastic leukemia. Blood Adv 2019;3(7):1039–46.

107. Hahn CN, Chong CE, Carmichael CL, et al. Heritable GATA2 mutations associated with familial myelodysplastic syndrome and acute myeloid leukemia. Nat Genet 2011;43(10):1012–7.

108. Hsu AP, Sampaio EP, Khan J, et al. Mutations in GATA2 are associated with the autosomal dominant and sporadic monocytopenia and mycobacterial infection (MonoMAC) syndrome. Blood 2011;118(10):2653–5.

109. Kazenwadel J, Secker GA, Liu YJ, et al. Loss-of-function germline GATA2 mutations in patients with MDS/AML or MonoMAC syndrome and primary lymphedema reveal a key role for GATA2 in the lymphatic vasculature. Blood 2012; 119(5):1283–91.

110. Spinner MA, Sanchez LA, Hsu AP, et al. GATA2 deficiency: a protean disorder of hematopoiesis, lymphatics, and immunity. Blood 2014;123(6):809–21.

111. Fisher KE, Hsu AP, Williams CL, et al. Somatic mutations in children with GATA2-associated myelodysplastic syndrome who lack other features of GATA2 deficiency. Blood Adv 2017;1(7):443–8.

112. Song WJ, Sullivan MG, Legare RD, et al. Haploinsufficiency of CBFA2 causes familial thrombocytopenia with propensity to develop acute myelogenous leukaemia. Nat Genet 1999;23(2):166–75.

113. Buijs A, Poddighe P, van Wijk R, et al. A novel CBFA2 single-nucleotide mutation in familial platelet disorder with propensity to develop myeloid malignancies. Blood 2001;98(9):2856–8.

114. Beri-Dexheimer M, Latger-Cannard V, Philippe C, et al. Clinical phenotype of germline RUNX1 haploinsufficiency: from point mutations to large genomic deletions. Eur J Hum Genet 2008;16(8):1014–8.

115. Owen CJ, Toze CL, Koochin A, et al. Five new pedigrees with inherited RUNX1 mutations causing familial platelet disorder with propensity to myeloid malignancy. Blood 2008;112(12):4639–45.

116. Sorrell A, Espenschied C, Wang W, et al. Hereditary leukemia due to rare RUNX1c splice variant (L472X) presents with eczematous phenotype. Int J Clin Med 2012;3(7):607–13.

117. Schmit JM, Turner DJ, Hromas RA, et al. Two novel RUNX1 mutations in a patient with congenital thrombocytopenia that evolved into a high grade myelodysplastic syndrome. Leuk Res Rep 2015;4(1):24–7.

118. Latger-Cannard V, Philippe C, Bouquet A, et al. Haematological spectrum and genotype-phenotype correlations in nine unrelated families with RUNX1 mutations from the French network on inherited platelet disorders. Orphanet J Rare Dis 2016;11:49.

119. Kanagal-Shamanna R, Loghavi S, DiNardo CD, et al. Bone marrow pathologic abnormalities in familial platelet disorder with propensity for myeloid malignancy and germline RUNX1 mutation. Haematologica 2017;102(10):1661–70.

120. Chisholm KM, Denton C, Keel S, et al. Bone marrow morphology associated with germline RUNX1 mutations in patients with familial platelet disorder with associated myeloid malignancy. Pediatr Dev Pathol 2019;22(4):315–28.

121. Chen DH, Below JE, Shimamura A, et al. Ataxia-pancytopenia syndrome is caused by missense mutations in SAMD9L. Am J Hum Genet 2016;98(6):1146–58.

122. Narumi S, Amano N, Ishii T, et al. SAMD9 mutations cause a novel multisystem disorder, MIRAGE syndrome, and are associated with loss of chromosome 7. Nat Genet 2016;48(7):792–7.

123. Buonocore F, Kuhnen P, Suntharalingham JP, et al. Somatic mutations and progressive monosomy modify SAMD9-related phenotypes in humans. J Clin Invest 2017;127(5):1700–13.

124. Sarthy J, Zha J, Babushok D, et al. Poor outcome with hematopoietic stem cell transplantation for bone marrow failure and MDS with severe MIRAGE syndrome phenotype. Blood Adv 2018;2(2):120–5.

125. Vlachos A, Rosenberg PS, Atsidaftos E, et al. Incidence of neoplasia in Diamond Blackfan anemia: a report from the Diamond Blackfan Anemia Registry. Blood 2012;119(16):3815–9.

126. Arbiv OA, Cuvelier G, Klaassen RJ, et al. Molecular analysis and genotype-phenotype correlation of Diamond-Blackfan anemia. Clin Genet 2018;93(2):320–8.

127. Simkins A, Bannon SA, Khoury JD, et al. Diamond-Blackfan anemia predisposing to myelodysplastic syndrome in early adulthood. JCO Precis Oncol 2017;(1):1–5.

128. Vlachos A, Rosenberg PS, Atsidaftos E, et al. Increased risk of colon cancer and osteogenic sarcoma in Diamond-Blackfan anemia. Blood 2018;132(20):2205–8.

129. Alter BP. Fanconi anemia and the development of leukemia. Best Pract Res Clin Haematol 2014;27(3–4):214–21.

130. Savage SA, Walsh MF. Myelodysplastic syndrome, acute myeloid leukemia, and cancer surveillance in Fanconi anemia. Hematol Oncol Clin North Am 2018;32(4):657–68.

131. Ayas M, Saber W, Davies SM, et al. Allogeneic hematopoietic cell transplantation for fanconi anemia in patients with pretransplantation cytogenetic abnormalities, myelodysplastic syndrome, or acute leukemia. J Clin Oncol 2013;31(13):1669–76.

132. Kutler DI, Singh B, Satagopan J, et al. A 20-year perspective on the International Fanconi Anemia Registry (IFAR). Blood 2003;101(4):1249–56.
133. Dokal I, Bungey J, Williamson P, et al. Dyskeratosis congenita fibroblasts are abnormal and have unbalanced chromosomal rearrangements. Blood 1992; 80(12):3090–6.
134. Yamaguchi H, Baerlocher GM, Lansdorp PM, et al. Mutations of the human telomerase RNA gene (TERC) in aplastic anemia and myelodysplastic syndrome. Blood 2003;102(3):916–8.
135. Ortmann CA, Niemeyer CM, Wawer A, et al. TERC mutations in children with refractory cytopenia. Haematologica 2006;91(5):707–8.
136. Armanios MY, Chen JJ, Cogan JD, et al. Telomerase mutations in families with idiopathic pulmonary fibrosis. N Engl J Med 2007;356(13):1317–26.
137. Kirwan M, Vulliamy T, Marrone A, et al. Defining the pathogenic role of telomerase mutations in myelodysplastic syndrome and acute myeloid leukemia. Hum Mutat 2009;30(11):1567–73.
138. Jyonouchi S, Forbes L, Ruchelli E, et al. Dyskeratosis congenita: a combined immunodeficiency with broad clinical spectrum–a single-center pediatric experience. Pediatr Allergy Immunol 2011;22(3):313–9.
139. Armanios M, Blackburn EH. The telomere syndromes. Nat Rev Genet 2012; 13(10):693–704.
140. Gorgy AI, Jonassaint NL, Stanley SE, et al. Hepatopulmonary syndrome is a frequent cause of dyspnea in the short telomere disorders. Chest 2015; 148(4):1019–26.
141. Stanley SE, Rao AD, Gable DL, et al. Radiation sensitivity and radiation necrosis in the short telomere syndromes. Int J Radiat Oncol Biol Phys 2015;93(5): 1115–7.
142. Burris AM, Ballew BJ, Kentosh JB, et al. Hoyeraal-Hreidarsson syndrome due to PARN mutations: fourteen years of follow-up. Pediatr Neurol 2016;56:62–68 e61.
143. Cardoso SR, Ellison ACM, Walne AJ, et al. Myelodysplasia and liver disease extend the spectrum of RTEL1 related telomeropathies. Haematologica 2017; 102(8):e293–6.
144. Wagner CL, Hanumanthu VS, Talbot CC Jr, et al. Short telomere syndromes cause a primary T cell immunodeficiency. The J Clin Invest 2018;128(12): 5222–34.
145. Donadieu J, Fenneteau O, Beaupain B, et al. Classification of and risk factors for hematologic complications in a French national cohort of 102 patients with Shwachman-Diamond syndrome. Haematologica 2012;97(9):1312–9.
146. Myers KC, Bolyard AA, Otto B, et al. Variable clinical presentation of Shwachman-Diamond syndrome: update from the North American Shwachman-Diamond Syndrome Registry. J Pediatr 2014;164(4):866–70.
147. Boocock GR, Morrison JA, Popovic M, et al. Mutations in SBDS are associated with Shwachman-Diamond syndrome. Nat Genet 2003;33(1):97–101.
148. Schlegelberger B, Kreipe H, Lehmann U, et al. A child with Li-Fraumeni syndrome: modes to inactivate the second allele of TP53 in three different malignancies. Pediatr Blood Cancer 2015;62(8):1481–4.
149. Swaminathan M, Bannon SA, Routbort M, et al. Hematologic malignancies and Li-Fraumeni syndrome. Cold Spring Harb Mol Case Stud 2019;5(1) [pii: a003210].
150. Talwalkar SS, Yin CC, Naeem RC, et al. Myelodysplastic syndromes arising in patients with germline TP53 mutation and Li-Fraumeni syndrome. Arch Pathol Lab Med 2010;134(7):1010–5.

151. Lynch HT, Weisenburger DD, Quinn-Laquer B, et al. Family with acute myelo-cytic leukemia, breast, ovarian, and gastrointestinal cancer. Cancer Genet Cy-togenet 2002;137(1):8–14.

152. Janiszewska H, Bak A, Skonieczka K, et al. Constitutional mutations of the CHEK2 gene are a risk factor for MDS, but not for de novo AML. Leuk Res 2018;70:74–8.

The Clinical Management of Clonal Hematopoiesis
Creation of a Clonal Hematopoiesis Clinic

Kelly L. Bolton, MD, PhD[a,c,*], Ahmet Zehir, PhD[b],
Ryan N. Ptashkin, MS[b], Minal Patel, MPH[c], Dipti Gupta, MD, MPH[d],
Robert Sidlow, MD, MBA[e], Elli Papaemmanuil, PhD[c,f],
Michael F. Berger, PhD[b,g,h], Ross L. Levine, MD[a,c,g]

KEYWORDS

- Clonal hematopoiesis • Clonal cytopenias of uncertain significance
- Clonal hematopoiesis of indeterminate significance

KEY POINTS

- The detection of acquired mutations in hematologic stem cells (clonal hematopoiesis) is common and can be identified as an incidental finding through clinical genetic testing.
- Clonal hematopoiesis is associated with a heightened risk of developing hematologic neoplasms (especially myeloid) and accelerated atherosclerotic cardiovascular disease.
- Patients with clonal hematopoiesis require a multidisciplinary clinical approach to management.

INTRODUCTION: CLONAL HEMATOPOIESIS IN THE CONTEXT OF NORMAL HUMAN AGING AND AS A PRECANCEROUS STATE

With every round of mitotic division, DNA damage and inefficient repair occur, resulting in the accumulation of somatic mutations in aging cells over time.[1] The development of somatic mutations in normal tissues has long been recognized as an aging

[a] Department of Medicine, Leukemia Service, Memorial Sloan Kettering Cancer Center, 1275 York Avenue, New York, NY 10065, USA; [b] Department of Pathology, Memorial Sloan Kettering Cancer Center, 1275 York Avenue, New York, NY 10065, USA; [c] Center for Hematologic Malignancies, Memorial Sloan Kettering Cancer Center, 1275 York Avenue, New York, NY 10065, USA; [d] Department of Medicine, Cardiology Service, Memorial Sloan Kettering Cancer Center, 1275 York Avenue, New York, NY 10065, USA; [e] Department of Medicine, General Internal Medicine Service, Memorial Sloan Kettering Cancer Center, 1275 York Avenue, New York, NY 10065, USA; [f] Department of Epidemiology and Biostatistics, Memorial Sloan Kettering Cancer Center, 1275 York Avenue, New York, NY 10065, USA; [g] Human Oncology & Pathogenesis Program, Memorial Sloan Kettering Cancer Center, 1275 York Avenue, New York, NY 10065, USA; [h] Marie-Josee and Henry R. Kravis Center for Molecular Oncology, Memorial Sloan Kettering Cancer Center, 1275 York Avenue, New York, NY 10065, USA
* Corresponding author.
E-mail address: boltonk@mskcc.org

Hematol Oncol Clin N Am 34 (2020) 357–367
https://doi.org/10.1016/j.hoc.2019.11.006
0889-8588/20/© 2019 Elsevier Inc. All rights reserved.

phenotype. With the advent of next-generation sequencing (NGS) technologies, an improved resolution has revealed that clonal expansion of cells with cancer-associated mutations are an extremely common, if not universal, condition in somatic tissues. Although somatic mutations are ubiquitous across a wide range of tissues, mutation rates and the spectra of driver genes differ among healthy tissues.[2–5] The former likely reflects a combination of tissue-specific intrinsic mutation rates[6] and environmental factors,[4] with the latter reflecting the importance of cellular context in mutation-induced differential fitness.[7] The overlap between the somatic mutation spectra of normal tissue and cancers in the same lineage suggests that the mutational processes operative in aging also underlie the development of cancer. Indeed, precancerous lesions can be identified in many tissue types that harbor similar mutations to their respective cancers.[8–10] Because of ease of sampling, somatic mutations in the blood have been the most frequently studied and are the focus of this article. The acquisition of somatic mutations leading to the clonal expansion of mutated hematopoietic cells is referred to as clonal hematopoiesis (CH). CH has gained considerable clinical interest because of its association with an increased risk of hematologic malignancies (especially myeloid neoplasms), shorter overall survival, and increased risk of cardiovascular disease (CVD).[11–16] This article first provides an overview of CH, including its epidemiology and relationship to hematologic malignancies and CVD risk. Following this overview, it describes the multitude of genomic profiling methods whereby CH can come to the attention of clinicians as an incidental finding. In addition, it describes the formation of a CH clinic at Memorial Sloan Kettering (MSK) Cancer Center and the current standard of practice for the clinical management of CH.

DEFINING CLONAL HEMATOPOIESIS

The first evidence of CH came from analysis of X-chromosome inactivation ratios in normal women that showed age-related skewing.[17] Since then, advances in genomics have revealed that CH is pervasive in aging populations. The prevalence of CH varies based on the age of the study population, sequencing methods, and the type of genetic alteration under investigation. Reports in the mid-1990s showed that gene fusions in BCR-ABL, associated with chronic myeloid leukemia and acute lymphoblastic leukemia, could be found at very low levels by polymerase chain reaction in healthy adults.[18] Analysis of single nucleotide polymorphism (SNP) arrays showed that clonal expansions of cells with large chromosome-level alterations could be detected in 0.5% of adults using standard analytical techniques for SNP arrays.[19,20] Subsequent reports indicate this is closer to 5% of adults when haplotype reconstruction methods for variant calling are used.[21] Analysis of whole-exome sequencing data from leukocyte-derived DNA showed age-dependent single nucleotide variants or small insertions/deletions in at least 6% of subjects more than 65 years of age.[11,13,22] Although mutations in more than 70 different genes were identified, the most frequently mutated genes were myeloid malignancy driver genes, including DNMT3A, TET2, and ASXL1. Error-correction NGS technologies have further improved the limit for mutation detection, and the prevalence of myeloid malignancy–associated mutations in the blood of adults more than 50 years old now seems closer to 100%.[23,24]

The term CH of indeterminate potential (CHIP) was coined by Steensma and colleagues[25] to describe CH at a variant allele fraction (VAF) greater than or equal to 2% in the absence of cytopenias in individuals without a hematologic malignancy. Age-related CH is a term used by some clinicians to emphasize that CH is a normal aging process that generally does not progress to hematologic malignancy. This article uses the more general term CH. Because a VAF of 2% is used in many current clinical sequencing assays as the cutoff for variant calling, this article defines CH as a somatic mutation in the peripheral blood at a VAF of 2%. However, the cutoff with clinical and biological significance remains to be delineated.

CLONAL HEMATOPOIESIS AND HEMATOLOGIC DISEASE

In 2014, three groups using analysis of whole-exome datasets from large cohorts of subjects showed that subjects with CH had a roughly 10-fold heightened risk of developing a hematological cancer, especially myeloid malignancies.[11,13,22] This risk of hematological malignancy was shown to increase with both the clone size (as measured by VAF) and the number of mutations.[11,13,22] However, these initial studies did not have sufficient power to study the strength of the association between CH in specific genes and hematologic cancer risk. Two recent studies performed targeted deep sequencing of the blood of healthy subjects drawn from large cohort studies in the United States and Europe who later developed acute myeloid leukemia (AML) and age-matched and sex-matched control groups of people who did not during the same follow-up period.[14,15] They showed that CH in specific genes confers particularly high risks of AML, including genes involved in pre–messenger RNA splicing (ie, spliceosome genes), *TP53* and *IDH1/2*.

In the general population, patients with CH and concurrent cytopenias are at high risk of occult myeloid neoplasms and ultimate development of overt hematologic malignancies.[26,27] It has been shown that cases of CH with a VAF greater than or equal to 10%, CH with multiple mutations, and spliceosome gene mutations have high positive predictive values (ranging from 0.86 to 1.0) for the presence of occult myeloid neoplasm among patients being evaluated for cytopenias.[27] Long-term follow-up of patients with a nondiagnostic bone marrow biopsy at initial evaluation showed that the presence of CH was highly predictive of the risk of transformation to hematologic malignancy (hazard ratio [HR], 13.9; 95% confidence interval [CI], 5.40–35.91; 5-year and 10-year cumulative probabilities of progression, 82% vs 9% and 95% vs 9% respectively; $P < .001$). This finding suggests that subsets of patients with CH and cytopenias are at a significantly higher risk for occult myeloid malignancy.

Patients with solid tumors of almost all primary tumor types are at a heightened risk for developing therapy-related myeloid neoplasm (tMN), including therapy-related AML and therapy-related myelodysplastic syndrome (MDS).[28] Therapy-related myeloid neoplasms represent up to 20% of new diagnoses of myeloid neoplasm and portend very poor prognosis (overall survival, 6–12 months). Takahasi and colleagues[29] and Gillis and colleagues[30] reported that a higher prevalence of CH at the time of primary (solid) cancer diagnosis has been observed in individuals who developed tMN compared with matched patients who did not develop tMN (62% vs 27%, $P = .02$; and 71% vs 31%, $P = .008$, respectively). These studies were not powered to discriminate the effects of individual genes or the association between blood count indexes and risk of tMN. Whether the relative strength of clinical and mutational features for myeloid malignancy risk will be similar in patients with solid tumors compared with healthy patients or distinct under the selective pressure of oncologic therapy has yet to be determined. However, given evidence that CH caused by mutations in specific genes (ie, *TP53*) shows a strong selective advantage in the specific context of oncologic therapy,[31] the risk for CH with mutations in specific genes is likely to be modified by exposure to therapy.

CH induced by large chromosome-level alterations have been associated with a 10-fold increased risk of developing a hematological cancer.[19,21] Unlike CH driven by point mutations or small insertions or deletions, large structural alterations show a stronger association with lymphoid malignancies, especially chronic lymphoid leukemia (CLL), compared with myeloid malignancies. This finding likely reflects a propensity toward chromosome-level early driver events in CLL (ie, del 13q, del 11q).[32]

CLONAL HEMATOPOIESIS AND CARDIOVASCULAR DISEASE

CH has been associated with an increased risk of CVD, including coronary heart disease (HR, 1.9; 95% CI, 1.4–2.7), ischemic stroke (HR, 2.6; 95% CI, 1.4–4.8), and early-onset myocardial infarction (HR, 4.0; 95% CI, 2.4–6.7).[11,12] The strength of the association between CH and CVD was comparable with well-validated traditional cardiovascular risk factors, such as high cholesterol, smoking, and hypertension. Individuals harboring the JAK2 V617F mutation had a particularly increased risk for CVD (HR, 12.0; 95% CI, 3.8–38.4).[12] As with the association between CH and risk of hematologic malignancy, the risk of incident coronary disease was shown to increase with higher clonal burden (HR, 2.2; 95% CI, 1.4–3.30 for VAF >10% and HR, 1.4; 95% CI, 0.9–2.4 for VAF <10%).

The mechanisms underlying the association between CH and CVD are in the early phases of being studied and are likely multifactorial. Murine studies show that genetically altered mice with reduced TET2 expression in hematopoietic cells, including monocytes/macrophages, develop accelerated atherosclerosis,[12,33] and heart failure[34]; these cardiac phenotypes are associated with increased macrophage activation and expression of the proinflammatory cytokine, interleukin (IL)-1β. This finding is echoed by human data linking TET2 CH to higher circulating levels of IL-8.[12,34] At present, there are no evidence-based approaches to reducing CH-associated CVD risk. Furthermore, the ability to generalize the mechanisms linking TET2 CH and CVD to the full spectrum of acquired mutations observed in CH is unknown.

DETECTION OF CLONAL HEMATOPOIESIS IN CLINICAL GENETIC ASSAYS

As genetic profiling is increasingly entering into clinical care, the possibility of incidental or systematic discovery of CH is increasingly likely. CH can be discovered incidentally when sequencing blood or saliva (because of infiltrating leukocytes) for the purpose of germline testing.[35,36] CH can be identified during the evaluation of unexplained cytopenias, frequently encountered in older adults. The National Comprehensive Cancer Network guidelines for MDS recommend sequencing of MDS-associated genes in patients with cytopenias when there is suspicion for MDS.[37] In a substantial proportion of patients with cytopenias, somatic mutations in malignancy-related genes are present, and, if the VAF of this clonal cell population is greater than or equal to 2%, this condition is described as clonal cytopenia of undetermined (or unknown) significance.[26,27,38] This population represents a group at particularly high risk for developing myeloid neoplasms, as previously described. In patients with cancer, in whom tumor sequencing is increasingly performed as standard practice, CH can be detected through several sources. First, when tumor sequencing is accompanied by blood sequencing as a patient-matched control, CH can be uncovered from the blood sequencing data as an incidental finding.[39] Second, CH can be discovered in tests of plasma cell-free DNA, much of which is derived from white blood cells and can confound these results aimed to reflect epithelial tumor genotypes.[40,41] Third, CH can be detected in tumor-only solid tumor sequencing because of blood contamination of tumor samples, leading to false-positive somatic mutation calls misattributed to the solid tumor.[42–44] In addition, in the setting of bone marrow transplant, CH can be transferred from donor to recipient and can be detected in standard assays for disease surveillance.[45] Thus, clinicians should be prepared to counsel and manage patients with CH.

MULTIDISCIPLINARY CLINICAL MANAGEMENT OF PATIENTS WITH CLONAL HEMATOPOIESIS

A review of the literature highlights the complexity of the relationship between CH, CVD, and hematologic malignancy and the rapid evolution of the field. Advances in sequencing technologies and analytical methods will provide increasing resolution to detect CH events and will both further elucidate and complicate the clinical implications of CH. In order to counsel patients regarding findings of CH, a multidisciplinary approach is required, including clinical practitioners and geneticists familiar with the field. Thus, the authors formed a CH clinic at MSK with dedicated providers and an established clinical work flow for the management of CH. At present, our CH clinic involves providers from hematology/oncology, cardiology, internal medicine, pathology, clinical genetics, and bioinformatics.

In the absence of evidence-based guidelines, this article discusses our general management strategies for individuals who have CH. When CH is detected as an incidental finding from blood DNA analysis, we do not systematically inform all individuals of CH because of the lack of established interventional strategies. When individuals are found to have CH and abnormal blood count indexes and/or high-risk mutational characteristics, such as a VAF greater than or equal to 10% and/or more than 1 mutation, especially in high-risk genes (*IDH1/2*, *TP53*, spliceosome gene class), we recommend that patients and their care teams be notified of the presence of CH in order to consider evaluation for an occult hematologic disorder. When discovered as an incidental finding in a patient with a solid tumor, we advise that the decision to further evaluate for CH should take into account the patient's prognosis and personal preferences. Because of the difficulty in discriminating CH from artifacts and germline variation, we confirm the presence of CH in the blood using our internal panel, MSK-IMPACT-Heme, using nails as a matched control. Details on our quality control, variant calling, and post-processing filters are described elsewhere.[39]

When CH is discovered during a work-up of cytopenias, we evaluate for alternative causes on history, physical, and laboratory results, such as iron deficiency anemia and anemia of chronic kidney disease. If no alternative cause for cytopenias is identified on initial work-up, a bone marrow biopsy is performed. Because of interobserver variability in MDS diagnosis, particularly MDS with unilineage dysplasia, bone marrow biopsies are reviewed by a hematopathologist specializing in MDS.[46] Quantification of dysplasia in all cell lineages is performed as part of pathology review. For individuals with CH who have no overt evidence of hematologic disease, we perform infrequent follow-up, including yearly monitoring of blood count indexes. For patients with abnormal blood counts, we repeat complete blood counts every 3 to 12 months, depending on the severity of blood count abnormalities. In patients who have progressive blood count abnormalities or other symptoms concerning for evolving hematologic disease, we repeat mutational testing and a bone marrow biopsy. When CH is discovered in patients with early-stage, surgically resected solid tumors who are considering adjuvant therapy, this poses a particular conundrum to oncologists. The risk of tMN must always be weighed against the benefit of decreased tumor recurrence rates when deciding whether to pursue adjuvant therapy. Although it is clear that patients with solid tumors with CH are at a heightened risk of tMN, an accurate quantification of this risk is not yet available. Although risk prediction models for AML in healthy individuals incorporating CH have been developed, the extent to which these can be extended to patients with solid tumors receiving systemic oncologic therapy and/or radiotherapy is unclear. Models integrating the impact of CH and past and future planned oncologic therapy on tMN risk have yet to be explored. Our general practice is to provide estimates on the absolute risk of tMN following the planned adjuvant therapy based on the literature and to counsel patients and oncologists that CH likely further increases this absolute risk of tMN. We emphasize in particular the potential for an increased risk of tMN following cytotoxic therapy in patients with preexisting *TP53* CH given evidence of therapy-induced expansion of *TP53* mutant hematopoietic stem cells (HSCs).[31,47]

To address the increased risk of CVD associated with CH, the authors offer all our patients with CH consultation with a cardiologist and/or primary care physician. At present, there is a lack of data and evidence-based recommendations targeted to decrease CH-associated cardiovascular risk; furthermore, it remains unaccounted for in the traditional cardiovascular risk models and, until such data are available, the preferred management strategy is individualized risk assessment and counseling to generate awareness among patients and mitigating the overall CV risk by using guideline-concordant primary and secondary cardiovascular prevention. We perform a thorough assessment of traditional cardiovascular risk factors, including tobacco use, family history of premature atherosclerotic CVD (ASCVD), hypertension, diabetes mellitus, chronic inflammatory diseases, and dyslipidemia. All patients undergo systolic and diastolic blood pressure measurement, physical examination (including body mass index), and a lipid panel including low-density lipoprotein, triglycerides, high-density lipoprotein, high-sensitivity C-reactive protein, hemoglobin A1c, and fasting glucose. We calculate 10-year risk and, when appropriate, the lifetime risk of heart disease or stroke using the ASCVD algorithm and use this to guide further nonpharmacologic and pharmacologic interventions per the American College of Cardiology (ACC)/American Heart Association (AHA) guidelines.[48] In patients at intermediate risk, computed tomography–derived coronary artery calcium score is often recommended to assess for subclinical atherosclerotic disease and aid in further risk stratification. We emphasize ACC/AHA lifestyle recommendations specifically to engage in at least 150 min/wk of accumulated moderate-intensity or 75 min/wk of vigorous-intensity aerobic physical activity (or an equivalent combination of moderate and vigorous activity). We encourage a heart-healthy diet, encouraging intake of vegetables, fruits and whole grains, low-fat dairy products, poultry, fish, legumes, nontropical vegetable oils and nuts, and limitation of sweets, sugar-sweetened beverages, and red meats. The use of aspirin in primary prevention has come under considerable scrutiny in light of recent clinical trials and we do not routinely recommend aspirin use in patients with CH.[49] The specific role of aspirin in primary prophylaxis in CH is particularly salient in patients with CH with *JAK2* V617F mutations, given their heightened risk of CVD and the established role of aspirin in thromboprophylaxis in myeloproliferative neoplasms. There is thus an imperative for clinical studies to address this critical question.

At present, there is a lack of data and evidence-based recommendations targeted to decrease CH-associated cardiovascular risk; furthermore, it remains unaccounted for in the traditional cardiovascular risk models and, until such data are available, the preferred management strategy is individualized risk assessment and counseling to generate awareness among patients and mitigating the overall CV risk by using guideline-concordant primary and secondary cardiovascular prevention.

FUTURE DIRECTIONS IN CLINICAL MANAGEMENT

Although ongoing research will lead to improved characterization of the adverse health outcomes associated with CH, interventional trials in patients with CH will be needed to transform the knowledge into clinical action. Crucially, it remains to be determined whether the incidence of CVD, hematologic malignancy, and other adverse health outcomes in individuals with CH will be reduced through preemptive treatment, although several promising approaches exist. The formation of CH clinics will be critical in achieving this. In addition to facilitating clinical care, CH clinics provide a foundation for recruiting individuals to participate in intervention trials designed to prevent hematologic malignancies and reduce the risk of CH-associated sequelae, including CVD.

The characterization of tumor genetic drivers, combined with an increasing understanding of the genetically driven tumor vulnerabilities, has led to the development of genome-driven precision therapies and combinatorial treatment approaches. Patients with cancer are benefiting from a diverse array of US Food and Drug Administration (FDA)–approved therapies targeting the somatic genetic aberrations in their tumors, and many of these therapies are FDA approved in the up-front setting.[50] The use of gene-specific targeted therapies early on, in the premalignant stage, has not yet been explored. Applying such therapies in the asymptomatic phase of CH might prevent further progression and development of myeloid neoplasms. However, as with preventive interventions in general, chemoprevention agents must be proved to be safe before their use can be justified in asymptomatic individuals, even in those at high risk. The use of genetically targeted therapies for myeloid disease is in its early stages, but promising candidates for mechanism-based clinical trials can already be identified, including IDH1[51] and IDH2[52] inhibitors. Prevention of the evolution of CH to overt neoplasia might also be possible through antiinflammatory therapies, which alter the fitness landscape by reducing systemic inflammation. A central role of chronic inflammation and oxidative stress in myeloid neoplasms has been posited, including its progression and clonal evolution from CH.[53] Preclinical evidence suggests that vitamin C can suppress TET2 mutant leukemic stem cell proliferation and leukemia progression through epigenetic modulation,[54,55] which in turn may ameliorate the proinflammatory effect of TET2 loss.[56] A clinical trial evaluating the safety and efficacy of high-dose vitamin C in the treatment of TET2-mutated MDS (NCT03433781) is ongoing and, if successful, will provide further rationale for investigating the use of antiinflammatory agents in CH.

Aggressive lifestyle modification and other traditional CVD preventive measures (ie, statins) could reduce CVD events in individuals with CH. As such, at MSK, we have an ongoing clinical trial regarding the use of intensive exercise training to both modify the natural history of CH (through clonal stabilization related to the antiinflammatory effects of exercise) and to reduce the incidence of CVD events (NCT01943695). The use of antiinflammatory treatments for prevention of primary and secondary CVD events, particularly in individuals with CH, is an exciting area of future research. The role of inflammation in human cardiovascular events has long been a vibrant area of investigation. Recently, a large prospective randomized clinical trial of canakinumab, an anti–IL-1β monoclonal antibody, versus placebo in patients with a prior myocardial infarction and persistently increased levels of the inflammatory marker C-reactive protein showed lower recurrent events in the intervention group.[57] Baseline samples from the patients in that study are being examined to see whether those with CH benefited most from the intervention. If so, this suggests a potential tool for reducing CVD in patients with CH. Although the FDA has not approved canakinumab for cardiovascular risk reduction, several other agents targeting inflammatory mediators are in development for CVD risk mitigation.

SUMMARY

Aging is accompanied by the accumulation of somatic mutations in healthy tissue, including HSCs giving rise in some cases to CH. Although CH can be considered a process of aging and is a common finding in genetic testing, its associations with adverse health outcomes, including CVD and hematologic malignancy, may warrant, in some cases, clinical counseling. CH clinics help facilitate the multidisciplinary care required for the management of patients with CH. Dedicated CH clinics will also facilitate interventional studies that may lead to improved outcomes for patients with CH and serve as a clinical platform for next-generation molecularly informed prevention strategies.

DISCLOSURE

A. Zehir has received honoraria from Illumina. M.F. Berger has consulted and served on the advisory board for Roche and has received research support from Illumina. R. Levine is on the supervisory board of Qiagen. He is a scientific advisor to Loxo, Imago, C4 Therapeutics, and Isoplexis, which includes equity interest. He receives research support from and has consulted for Celgene and Roche. He has consulted for Lilly, Janssen, Astellas, Morphosys, and Novartis. He has received honoraria from Roche, Lilly, Amgen, and Gilead.

REFERENCES

1. López-Otín C, Blasco MA, Partridge L, et al. The hallmarks of aging. Cell 2013; 153:1194–217.
2. Martincorena I, Fowler JC, Wabik A, et al. Somatic mutant clones colonize the human esophagus with age. Science 2018;362:911–7.
3. Martincorena I, Raine KM, Gerstung M, et al. Universal patterns of selection in cancer and somatic tissues. Cell 2018;173:1823.
4. Martincorena I, Roshan A, Gerstung M, et al. Tumor evolution. High burden and pervasive positive selection of somatic mutations in normal human skin. Science 2015;348:880–6.
5. Blokzijl F, de Ligt J, Jager M, et al. Tissue-specific mutation accumulation in human adult stem cells during life. Nature 2016;538:260–4.
6. Tomasetti C, Vogelstein B. Cancer etiology. Variation in cancer risk among tissues can be explained by the number of stem cell divisions. Science 2015;347:78–81.
7. Hart T, Chandrashekhar M, Aregger M, et al. High-resolution CRISPR screens reveal fitness genes and genotype-specific cancer liabilities. Cell 2015;163: 1515–26.
8. Anglesio MS, Papadopoulos N, Ayhan A, et al. Cancer-associated mutations in endometriosis without cancer. N Engl J Med 2017;376:1835–48.
9. Fearon ER. Molecular genetics of colorectal cancer. Annu Rev Pathol 2011;6: 479–507.
10. Martelotto LG, Baslan T, Kendall J, et al. Whole-genome single-cell copy number profiling from formalin-fixed paraffin-embedded samples. Nat Med 2017;23: 376–85.
11. Jaiswal S, Fontanillas P, Flannick J, et al. Age-related clonal hematopoiesis associated with adverse outcomes. N Engl J Med 2014;371:2488–98.
12. Jaiswal S, Natarajan P, Silver AJ, et al. Clonal hematopoiesis and risk of atherosclerotic cardiovascular disease. New Engl J Med 2017;377:111–21.

13. Genovese G, Kähler AK, Handsaker RE, et al. Clonal hematopoiesis and blood-cancer risk inferred from blood DNA sequence. N Engl J Med 2014;371:2477–87.
14. Abelson S, Collord G, Ng SWK, et al. Prediction of acute myeloid leukaemia risk in healthy individuals. Nature 2018;559:400–4.
15. Desai P, Mencia-Trinchant N, Savenkov O, et al. Somatic mutations precede acute myeloid leukemia years before diagnosis. Nat Med 2018;24:1015–23.
16. Young AL, Tong RS, Birmann BM, et al. Clonal haematopoiesis and risk of acute myeloid leukemia. Haematologica 2019. https://doi.org/10.3324/haematol.2018.215269.
17. Busque L, Mio R, Mattioli J, et al. Nonrandom X-inactivation patterns in normal females: lyonization ratios vary with age. Blood 1996;88:59–65.
18. Bose S, Deininger M, Gora-Tybor J, et al. The presence of typical and atypical BCR-ABL fusion genes in leukocytes of normal individuals: biologic significance and implications for the assessment of minimal residual disease. Blood 1998;92:3362–7.
19. Jacobs KB, Yeager M, Zhou W, et al. Detectable clonal mosaicism and its relationship to aging and cancer. Nat Genet 2012;44:651–8.
20. Laurie CC, Laurie CA, Rice K, et al. Detectable clonal mosaicism from birth to old age and its relationship to cancer. Nat Genet 2012;44:642–50.
21. Loh P-R, Genovese G, Handsaker RE, et al. Insights into clonal haematopoiesis from 8,342 mosaic chromosomal alterations. Nature 2018;559:350–5.
22. Xie M, Lu C, Wang J, et al. Age-related mutations associated with clonal hematopoietic expansion and malignancies. Nat Med 2014;20:1472–8.
23. Young AL, Challen GA, Birmann BM, et al. Clonal haematopoiesis harbouring AML-associated mutations is ubiquitous in healthy adults. Nat Commun 2016;7:12484.
24. Krimmel JD, Schmitt MW, Harrell MI, et al. Ultra-deep sequencing detects ovarian cancer cells in peritoneal fluid and reveals somatic TP53 mutations in noncancerous tissues. Proc Natl Acad Sci U S A 2016;113:6005–10.
25. Steensma DP, Bejar R, Jaiswal S, et al. Clonal hematopoiesis of indeterminate potential and its distinction from myelodysplastic syndromes. Blood 2015;126:9–16.
26. Kwok B, Hall JM, Witte JS, et al. MDS-associated somatic mutations and clonal hematopoiesis are common in idiopathic cytopenias of undetermined significance. Blood 2015;126:2355–61.
27. Malcovati L, Gallì A, Travaglino E, et al. Clinical significance of somatic mutation in unexplained blood cytopenia. Blood 2017;129:3371–8.
28. Morton LM, Dores GM, Tucker MA, et al. Evolving risk of therapy-related acute myeloid leukemia following cancer chemotherapy among adults in the United States, 1975-2008. Blood 2013;121:2996–3004.
29. Takahashi K, Wang F, Kantarjian H, et al. Preleukaemic clonal haemopoiesis and risk of therapy-related myeloid neoplasms: a case-control study. Lancet Oncol 2017;18:100–11.
30. Gillis NK, Ball M, Zhang Q, et al. Clonal haemopoiesis and therapy-related myeloid malignancies in elderly patients: a proof-of-concept, case-control study. Lancet Oncol 2017;18:112–21.
31. Wong TN, Miller CA, Jotte MRM, et al. Cellular stressors contribute to the expansion of hematopoietic clones of varying leukemic potential. Nat Commun 2018;9:455.
32. Landau DA, Tausch E, Taylor-Weiner AN, et al. Mutations driving CLL and their evolution in progression and relapse. Nature 2015;526:525–30.

33. Fuster JJ, MacLauchlan S, Zuriaga MA, et al. Clonal hematopoiesis associated with TET2 deficiency accelerates atherosclerosis development in mice. Science 2017;355(6327):842–7.

34. Sano S, Oshima K, Wang Y, et al. Tet2-mediated clonal hematopoiesis accelerates heart failure through a mechanism involving the IL-1β/NLRP3 inflammasome. J Am Coll Cardiol 2018;71:875–86.

35. Coffee B, Cox HC, Kidd J, et al. Detection of somatic variants in peripheral blood lymphocytes using a next generation sequencing multigene pan cancer panel. Cancer Genet 2017;211:5–8.

36. Hinds DA, Barnholt KE, Mesa RA, et al. Germ line variants predispose to both JAK2 V617F clonal hematopoiesis and myeloproliferative neoplasms. Blood 2016;128:1121–8.

37. Greenberg PL, Stone RM, Al-Kali A, et al. Myelodysplastic syndromes, version 2.2017, NCCN clinical practice guidelines in oncology. J Natl Compr Canc Netw 2017;15:60–87.

38. Bejar R. CHIP, ICUS, CCUS and other four-letter words. Leukemia 2017;31: 1869–71.

39. Coombs CC, Zehir A, Devlin SM, et al. Therapy-related clonal hematopoiesis in patients with non-hematologic cancers is common and associated with adverse clinical outcomes. Cell Stem Cell 2017;21:374–82.e4.

40. Hu Y, Ulrich BC, Supplee J, et al. False-positive plasma genotyping due to clonal hematopoiesis. Clin Cancer Res 2018;24:4437–43.

41. Strickler JH, Loree JM, Ahronian LG, et al. Genomic landscape of cell-free DNA in patients with colorectal cancer. Cancer Discov 2018;8:164–73.

42. Severson EA, Riedlinger GM, Connelly CF, et al. Detection of clonal hematopoiesis of indeterminate potential in clinical sequencing of solid tumor specimens. Blood 2018;131:2501–5.

43. Ptashkin RN, Mandelker DL, Coombs CC, et al. Prevalence of clonal hematopoiesis mutations in tumor-only clinical genomic profiling of solid tumors. JAMA Oncol 2018;4:1589.

44. Coombs CC, Gillis NK, Tan X, et al. Identification of clonal hematopoiesis mutations in solid tumor patients undergoing unpaired next-generation sequencing assays. Clin Cancer Res 2018;24:5918–24.

45. Frick M, Chan W, Arends CM, et al. Role of donor clonal hematopoiesis in allogeneic hematopoietic stem-cell transplantation. J Clin Oncol 2019;37:375–85.

46. Font P, Ramsingh G, Young AL, et al. Interobserver variance in myelodysplastic syndromes with less than 5 % bone marrow blasts: unilineage vs. multilineage dysplasia and reproducibility of the threshold of 2 % blasts. Ann Hematol 2015; 94:565–73.

47. Wong TN, Ramsingh G, Young AL, et al. Role of TP53 mutations in the origin and evolution of therapy-related acute myeloid leukaemia. Nature 2015;518:552–5.

48. Arnett DK, Khera A, Blumenthal RS. 2019 ACC/AHA guideline on the primary prevention of cardiovascular disease: part 1, lifestyle and behavioral factors. JAMA Cardiol 2019. https://doi.org/10.1001/jamacardio.2019.2604.

49. Raber I, McCarthy CP, Vaduganathan M, et al. The rise and fall of aspirin in the primary prevention of cardiovascular disease. Lancet 2019;393:2155–67.

50. Hyman DM, Taylor BS, Baselga J. Implementing genome-driven oncology. Cell 2017;168:584–99.

51. DiNardo CD, Stein EM, de Botton S, et al. Durable remissions with ivosidenib in IDH1-mutated relapsed or refractory AML. N Engl J Med 2018;378:2386–98.

52. Stein EM, DiNardo CD, Pollyea DA, et al. Enasidenib in mutant IDH2 relapsed or refractory acute myeloid leukemia. Blood 2017;130:722–31.
53. Craver BM, El Alaoui K, Scherber RM, et al. The critical role of inflammation in the pathogenesis and progression of myeloid malignancies. Cancers (Basel) 2018; 10 [pii:E104].
54. Agathocleous M, Meacham CE, Burgess RJ, et al. Ascorbate regulates haematopoietic stem cell function and leukaemogenesis. Nature 2017;549:476–81.
55. Cimmino L, Dolgalev I, Wang Y, et al. Restoration of TET2 function blocks aberrant self-renewal and leukemia progression. Cell 2017;170:1079–95.e20.
56. Zhang Q, Zhao K, Shen Q, et al. Tet2 is required to resolve inflammation by recruiting Hdac2 to specifically repress IL-6. Nature 2015;525:389–93.
57. Ridker PM, Everett BM, Thuren T, et al. Antiinflammatory therapy with canakinumab for atherosclerotic disease. N Engl J Med 2017;377:1119–31.

Novel Prognostic Models for Myelodysplastic Syndromes

Jacob Shreve, MD, MS[a], Aziz Nazha, MD[b],*

KEYWORDS

• MDS • Model • Mutations

KEY POINTS

- Myelodysplastic syndromes have a heterogeneous clinical presentation, and properly stratifying patients according to predicted disease severity is integral to therapeutic decision making.
- Currently used risk-stratification systems assess traditional clinical features, such as the results from simple blood tests, peripheral blood smears, bone marrows biopsies, and cytogenetic data, and can underestimate of overestimate the risk in a subset of patients.
- Emerging risk-stratification models that incorporate large-scale genomic data with traditional features may allow more personalized disease prediction for individual patients.

INTRODUCTION

Myelodysplastic syndromes (MDS) comprise 1 of 5 major myeloid neoplasms[1] and are due to clonal myelopoiesis resulting in bone marrow dysplasia. MDS are commonly associated with cytopenias, but the extent of clinical presentation can vary significantly, from relatively benign with minimal or no intervention needed, to refractory to all treatment with quick progression to acute myeloid leukemia.[2] This variable clinical manifestation poses a particular challenge to providers when counseling patients about prognosis and choosing an appropriate treatment regimen, because overall survival (OS) is highly dependent on early risk stratification and therapeutic choice.[3–6] If risk stratification determines a patient to be low to intermediate risk by the revised International Prognostic Scoring System (IPSS-R), intervention largely involves anemia amelioration via transfusions and erythropoiesis stimulation with a concentration on quality of life.[3] Conversely, if a patient is found to be IPSS-R high risk, aggressive therapy involving hypomethylating agents (HMA), clinical trials, or stem cell transplantation should be initiated immediately, with the goal of improving OS.[6] This dichotomy in

[a] Department of Hematology and Medical Oncology, Cleveland Clinic, Taussig Cancer Center, Desk R35, 9500 Euclid Avenue, Cleveland, OH 44195, USA; [b] Department of Hematology and Medical Oncology, Cleveland Clinic, Center for Clinical Artificial Intelligence, Lerner College of Medicine, Case Western Reserve University, Taussig Cancer Institute, Desk R35, 9500 Euclid Avenue, Cleveland, OH 44195, USA
* Corresponding author.
E-mail address: nazhaa@ccf.org

Hematol Oncol Clin N Am 34 (2020) 369–378
https://doi.org/10.1016/j.hoc.2019.10.001
0889-8588/20/© 2019 Elsevier Inc. All rights reserved.

treatment underlines the importance of accurate risk stratification at the time of diagnosis: a middle-aged man with low-risk disease may be treated conservatively without the use curative stem cell transplant and enjoy a high quality of life with good prognosis, but if his low-risk status was misassigned, conservative therapy would dramatically reduce his survival.

Risk stratification for MDS patients has been a dominant research target for many years, with numerous prognostic models proposed, the most common of which is the IPSS and the IPSS-R.[4,7–10] Such models rely on traditional clinical features, such as results from standard blood tests, peripheral smears, bone marrow biopsies, and cytogenetics, which when analyzed together, create a useful but imperfect representation of a patient's disease status. New technologies have allowed a far more precise genomic analysis of MDS, revealing a complicated interplay of traditional features with specific genetic markers, yielding a new generation of genomic-clinical prognostic modeling that is still in its infancy.[11–13]

Here, the authors evaluate the state of MDS risk-stratification systems in the clinic, discuss current efforts to increase the precision of such systems via hybridization with genomic data, and outline the expected developmental trajectory of MDS personalized prediction models.

MYELODYSPLASTIC SYNDROMES CLINICAL PROGNOSTIC MODELS

Current MDS clinical prognostic models rely on a combination of patient-related factors and disease-related factors to make disease severity predictions (**Fig. 1**). Patient-related factors include intrinsic attributes, such as age and sex, as well as measurements of performance status and comorbidities, such as heart failure, chronic kidney disease, and cirrhosis. Disease-related factors are divided into pathologic classifications using defined scoring systems, clinical variables obtained through standard laboratory testing, and biological variables, such as cytogenetics, DNA sequencing, and other omic-scale technologies. The interaction of the numerous patient-related factors and disease-related factors is untenably complex, and no current model includes all available factors. In addition, the factors interact in nonlinear ways, with certain factors

Patient-Related	Disease-Related
• Age	• Clinical variables
• Performance status	• Hemoglobin • Platelets
• Frailty	• White blood cell count • Absolute neutrophil count
• Comorbidities	• Blast percentage • LDH
• Renal	• Ferritin
• Cardiac	• Albumin
• Pulmonary	• Biological variables
• Others	• Cytogenetics • DNA sequencing
	• RNA Sequencing • Methylation profile
	• MicroRNA • Others
	• 2016 WHO Classification
	• Flow Cytometry

Fig. 1. Prognostic factors in MDS. Prognostic factors can be largely divided into patient-related and disease-related groupings, with several subgroups thereafter. LDH, lactate dehydrogenase.

potentiating and modifying others. For example, a patient diagnosed with refractory anemia with excess blasts-1 will likely have significantly different cytopenias and clinical outcomes if cytogenetic analysis identifies high-risk features rather than low-risk features. Because of current modeling limitations, current prognostic systems at use in the clinical and in clinical trial eligibility depend on mostly clinical variables.

MDS prognostic scoring systems have been the subject of research for many years, the most commonly used of which include the World Health Organization (WHO) Prognostic Scoring System (WPSS), the Global MD Anderson Prognostic Scoring System (MDAPSS), IPSS, and IPSS-R.[7–9,14,15] Despite the diversity of originating development teams, each of these models uses the same 3 broad factors to drive prognostic scoring: cytopenias (either directly measured from laboratory tests or indirectly as transfusion dependency, such as in WPSS), bone marrow blast percentage (although WPSS again uses an indirect assessment, namely WHO classification), and cytogenetic classification. IPSS-R-age and MDAPSS include age as an independent prognostic factor, whereas the remaining models only indirectly evaluate age by assessing other factors. IPSS and IPSS-R enjoy the most widespread use by clinicians to guide both treatment decisions and trial eligibility but are imperfect and do miscategorize a significant subset of patients because of a lack of complexity and factor utilization, and possibly because of pitfalls in model design.

Applying Prognostic Models in Patients with Therapy-Related or Secondary Myelodysplastic Syndromes

Although the IPSS and IPSS-R models were validated in both patients receiving lenalidomide, an HMA, and in those who went on to undergo hemopoietic cell transplantation (HCT), the algorithms were originally designed using pretreatment, de novo patients with MDS[8,16] and have not been found to be predictive of patient outcomes in cases of therapy-related or secondary MDS.[17–19]

Models Lack Dynamicity and Are Unable to Accommodate Hypomethylating Treatment Failure

MDS prognosis evolves after the time of diagnosis because of shifting patient-related and disease-related factors. An ideal model would be applicable at any time during the disease's progression and would be used to determine the best course of action during each clinical development. The models considered here were designed using factors obtained at the time of diagnosis and were validated at time points later in the disease progression but only for patients who did not receive disease-modifying treatment. For those patients who did receive HMA and particularly for those who failed treatment, these models have not been validated.[15] This is illustrated by an example in which a patient has a low-risk classification as per IPSS but undergoes 6 cycles of HMA treatment and fails to respond. This patient's OS is unchanged under current scoring systems and has a predicted OS of 5.7 years, but patients belonging to this cohort have been empirically demonstrated to have a median OS of 4 to 6 months.[20–22] Despite these shortcomings, IPSS and IPSS-R are still used for risk stratification by most clinical trials that assess alternative therapy after failing HMA. To better predict prognosis after HMA failure, a new model was created using age, performance status, platelet count, marrow blast percentage, transfusion dependence, and cytogenetics (**Table 1**). This model can classify patients as either low risk or high risk with predicted OS of 11.0 months (95% confidence interval [CI] 8.8–13.6) and 4.5 months (95% CI 3.9–5.3), respectively.[23] This model was validated on MDS patients in data from a prospective trial (n = 223, from the Groupe Francophone des Myélodysplasies), which

Table 1
Post hypomethylating agents failure model

Parameter at HMA Failure	Score
ECOG performance status >1	1.0
Complex karyotype ($\geq$4 abnormalities)	1.0
Age, years	
>75–$\leq$84	1.0
>84	2.0
Bone marrow blast >20%	.75
Transfusion dependent (yes)	.75
Platelets $\times$ 10^9/L	
<30	1.0

Risk	Score	Median OS
Lower	$\leq$2.25	11.0 mo
Higher	>2.25	4.5 mo

Abbreviation: ECOG, Eastern Cooperative Oncology Group.

compared rigosertib therapy to supportive care retrospectively in clinical data from patients treated in the French registry.[13,24]

Intermediate Risk Confusion

The IPSS model was by far the most commonly used model before the IPSS-R construct and would risk-stratify patients into low-, intermediate-1, intermediate-2, or high-risk cohorts, with low and intermediate-1 patients generally comprising the low-risk group, and the intermediate-2 and high patients comprising the high-risk group. However, the IPSS-R model unified intermediate-1 and -2 into a single intermediate group. Clinical trials have struggled to decide if intermediate patients should be considered in the low-risk or high-risk cohorts because IPSS-R intermediate patients have a variety of outcomes. An additional study determined an IPSS-R score cutoff of 3.5 points could divide patients between low-risk and high-risk disease.[10] Similarly, low-risk patients may be at exaggerated risk for aggressive transformation and should therefore be considered high risk if they possess aberrations of ferritin or lactate dehydrogenase or have certain mutations (namely *EXH2* or *TP53*).[25]

Risk Estimation Discrepancies

All prognostic models currently available suffer from risk-assignment discrepancies that cause inaccurate OS prediction for a sizable number of patients. For example, 25% to 30% of patients identified as lower risk by the IPSS model would be classified as higher risk by the MD Anderson Lower Risk Prognostic Scoring System (LRPSS) and would have predicted OS similar to that as IPSS higher-risk patients. The LRPSS model makes predictions by considering age, thrombocytopenia, bone marrow blast percentage, severity of anemia, and cytogenetic features.[7] Additional evidence that significant risk estimation discrepancies exist between all available models can be appreciated when considering a cohort of 687 MDS patients from Cleveland Clinic.[26] These patients demonstrated substantial differences between predicted and actual OS regardless of the model used. Consider the difference between mean IPSS-R predicted and measured OS for the following risk categories: 70.6 months for very low risk, 54 months for low risk, 9.5 months for intermediate risk, 6.7 months for high risk, and −2.4 months for very high risk. IPSS-R dramatically overestimated OS in less severe cases. The difference becomes less pronounced with increasingly severe risk stratification owing to the diminished likely window of survival, but it is notable that the actual OS was longer than predicted for the very high-risk category.[26] Conversely, the IPSS model underestimates OS: −23.3 months for low risk, −16.5 months for intermediate-1 risk, −11.8 months for intermediate-2 risk, and −11.1 months for high risk.[26] Such changes in predicted outcomes between 2 versions of the same model, both widely used clinically at different times, highlights the need to better predict prognosis because therapeutic choices are often directly made using this information.

MYELODYSPLASTIC SYNDROMES PROGNOSIS ALTERED BY SOMATIC MUTATIONS

In a departure from the traditional clinical features and cytogenetics used to understand MDS and its prognosis, a new wave of in-depth genomic analysis has revealed an abundance of variation seemingly correlated with disease severity, including several somatic mutations present in most patients.[11,27] Defining the compendium of common MDS-associated mutations has great implications in patient care, given that several mutations have been demonstrated to affect disease phenotype and severity, and therefore, prognosis.[11,27,28] Genomic data represent a new category from which disease-related factors can be defined and folded into the complex model of MDS pathology, and with the post–next-generation sequencing market allowing affordable large-scale sequencing, clinical assessment, and management of MDS may evolve to become increasingly genomics driven.

Myelodysplastic Syndromes Prognosis and Single Mutations

Several specific mutations have been identified that strongly correlate with OS, some of the most prominent of which include *EZH2*, *RUNX1*, *SF3B1*, and *TP53*.[11,12,25,27,28] Numerous other mutations have a more ambiguous effect on OS, including *DNMT3A*, *SRSF2*, *TET2*, and *U2AF1*.[11,12,25,27,28] These single mutations may have a less robust direct correlation to OS owing to an intrinsic complexity of gene interaction but also because of study-specific factors, such as population size and severity of MDS therein, in which genes were considered in the analysis, the tools used for the analysis, and other deviations that make mutation-effect generalizations difficult. Supporting this assessment, 1 study that considered 104 genes among 944 MDS patients found that 25 of 48 mutations were associated with reduced OS (including *ASXL1*, *EZH2*, *FLT3*, *GATA2*, *KRAS*, *LAMB4*, *LUC7L2*, *NF1*, *NPM1*, *NRAS*, *PRPF8*, *PTPN11*, *RUNX1*, *SMC1A*, and *TP53*), and only a single mutation was associated with increased OS (*SF3B1*).[11] Tellingly, of those 25 mutations, only 5 held significance after differentiating from clinical factors strongly associated with outcomes (*ASXL1*, *KRAS*, *PRPF8*, *RUNX1*, and *SF3B1*).[11] Similarly, another study involving 3562 MDS patients found a similar set of single mutations that were correlated with OS (*ASXL1*, *CBL*, *EZH2*, *KRAS*, *IDH2*, *NPM1*, *NRAS*, *RUNX1*, *SF3B1*, *TET2*, and *TP52*) if assessed through univariate analysis.[28] Defining which mutations independently modify OS is made significantly more difficult by clinical factors, which can dramatically alter the predictive nature of those mutations.[28] Consider a subset of genes that when mutated have been found to negatively modify OS (*ASXL1*, *SRSF2*, and *U2AF1*), but this effect is only significant when a patient's blast percentage is less than 5%; if greater, these mutations are no longer predictive. Again demonstrating the effect of clinical factor modulation, a study of 3392 patients and 27 genes found 12 mutations associated with shortened OS via univariate analysis, but after adjusting for the hazard ratio of death assigned by IPSS-R risk stratification, only 4 of those mutations were independently strong predictors of shortened OS.[28] The IPSS-R scoring system does not directly use several clinical factors known to correlate with OS, such as age, and therefore, the mutations found to be independently significant when adjusted to IPSS-R may require additional investigation.

Myelodysplastic Syndromes Prognosis and Intramutation Heterogeneity

Adding to the complexity of applying genomic analysis to MDS prognostic models, intramutational variation needs to be considered as well when measuring effect on OS. Current studies overwhelmingly evaluate mutations as discrete present or absent features, but the type of mutation (for example, missense vs nonsense), location of the mutation within the gene, and the variant allele frequency (VAF) should all be accounted for when considering if a mutation causes change to OS. Consider a study that attempts to determine if a particular mutated gene is associated with worse outcomes; if the population of "mutated" individuals in the analysis includes a subset of mutations in an important functional domain, as well as another subset with a minor missense mutation that does not interfere with protein folding or activity, the statistical significance of any conclusions will be skewed. Applying this to real-world MDS genomics, having a TP53 mutation is strongly associated with worse outcomes, but having a TP53 VAF of less than 25% (median OS 12.4 months) confers much less harm than a VAF of greater than 50% (median OS 3.4 months).[29] Understanding such intramutational heterogeneity will allow for more precise prognostic modeling.

Effect of Therapy on Mutation Prognostic Factors

Another consideration when determining if a mutation alters OS is the history of therapeutics in the patient being evaluated, because some interventions have been found to change prognostic mutations' significance. For example, there is contention regarding the prognostic ability of mutations after transplant.[30-33] Again using TP53 as an example, 1 study of 1514 patients found that the presence of a mutated copy was associated with poor outcomes despite correction for known clinical features.[34] Furthermore, intramutational heterogeneity was assessed, revealing worse outcomes with nonsense mutations and no impact if VAF was less than 10%.[34] The same study determined that patients with wild-type TP53 and who were at least 40 years old had decreased OS if mutations existed within the RAS pathway (CBL, FLT3, KIT, KRAS, NF1, NRAS, PTPN11, RIT1) because of increased chance of relapse, and decreased OS if JAK2 was mutated but without relapse.[34] In an analogous study using data from the Japanese bone marrow registry, decreased OS was associated with specific mutations (CBL, NRAS, and TP53) and with possessing a complex karyotype (CK).[33] These findings were independently significant even after correcting for clinical factors, but the OS-modulatory effect of TP53 was most prevalent in the CK cohort; without the CK attribute, TP53-mutated patients enjoyed better outcomes after transplant with 73% of patients still living 5 years after the procedure.[33] Again, the varying conclusions of these somewhat overlapping studies are mostly a result of different patient populations, inclusion of different clinical features, and different analysis methods. Although these studies demonstrate how TP53 can affect OS after the transplant, other treatment choices rather than HCT, such as the use of HMAs, were not evaluated. This fact is notable because some medicine-refractory TP53-mutated patients can improve OS with HCT, whereas others are unresponsive to HCT and have a very poor prognosis.

Prognostication with Mutations, Clinical Factors, or Both?

Historical risk-stratifying models relying on only clinical factors were improved once mutations highly associated with OS were included in the algorithm, and as more genomic analyses were conducted, a growing list of independently predictive mutations was discovered. Now the future of MDS prognostication needs to be considered, whether effort should be given toward refining clinically anchored models, developing mutation-only models, or creating a hybrid model that considers all available information. Clearly the predictive strength of certain mutations warrants inclusion, but as previously described, even the most influential mutations are subject to confounding clinical factors that create a whole new dimension of modeling complexity. Recent advancements attempting to combine traditional and genomic features into a model blended 14 mutations along with clinical variables similar to those found in the IPSS-R classification schema, including age and gender.[11] The hybrid genomic-clinical algorithm more accurately modeled MDS prognosis than either IPSS-R or a mutation-only model, which had similar results to each other.[11]

Intuitively and in practice, hybrid models that benefit from an increasing abundance of genomic data outperform models without mutational features, leading to much investigation into how best to combine these factors. A recent study on 508 patients from the Cleveland Clinic identified 6 mutations that shortened OS (ASXL1, EZH2, NPM1, RUNX1, and TP53) and one that that increased it (SF3B1).[12] Being part of a hybrid genomic-clinical model, other factors were included, but multivariate analysis only identified 5 total features to be significant: IPSS-R score, age, and the mutations EZH2, SF3B1, and TP53.[12] The significant features were then transformed into a linear algorithm using the prognostic factors' beta-coefficients, (Age $\times$ 0.04) + (IPSS-R score $\times$ 0.3) + (EZH2 $\times$ 0.7) + (SF3B1 $\times$ 0.5) + (TP53 $\times$ 1), and yielded a higher C-index than the IPSS-R scoring system. This hybrid system also made progress regarding MDS scoring systems' lack of dynamicity, with paired samples spanning different stages of disease progression able to be modeled.[12]

Spurred by the early success of genomic-clinical hybrid models, another Cleveland Clinic study of 610 patients used univariate analysis to determine 5 familiar gene mutations that correlated with OS (EZH2, NPM1, RUNX1, SF3B1, and TP53) and then reduced the number to 3 mutations after adjusting for age and model scores (EZH2, SF3B1, TP53).[25] These high-confidence OS-modifying mutations combined with age and added to the most commonly used preexisting MDS prognostic models. Every model assessed not only had improved prognostic ability but also reassigned many patient risk classifications, increasing accuracy. IPSS-R, in particular, being the most widely used model by practitioners today, had 26% of patients reassigned from the low-risk category to the high-risk category, along with 62% of the patients in the intermediate-risk category.[25]

A Goal of Personalized Prognostication

Management of the MDS patient requires early prognostication to guide patient expectations, therapy selection, and ultimately, OS, which emphasizes the shortcomings of currently used models that frequently misassign patient risk stratification. As demonstrated previously, work toward a genomic-clinical hybrid model increases accuracy of risk assignment and moves closer to personalized prediction. However, the complexity of molecular interaction with clinical variables both at the time of diagnosis and evolving throughout the disease course demands a modernized, more sophisticated statistical algorithm. To accomplish such a task, machine learning may take the place of traditional Cox regression analysis, allowing for more complex variable interactions and random selection of features to use for OS prediction.[32] In a multicenter study of 2302 patients with MDS, variable importance analysis revealed several key clinical and mutational features that strongly contribute to OS,[32] advancing the model's prognostic accuracy even beyond that of all established clinical scoring systems despite mutational data added. These promising preliminary results are currently being validated with a multinational dataset to demonstrate universal efficacy and will be delivered to clinicians via Web interface to facilitate experimentation and adaptation. This well-hybridized model that allows for clinical and molecular data to interact in unsupervised, unpredictable ways brings MDS risk stratification closer to truly personalized prognostication and may be applicable in other cancers as well.

SUMMARY

The current state of MDS therapy relies heavily on early prognostic stratification to guide patient expectations and choice of intervention. Traditional scoring systems in widespread use today are based on clinical features, cytogenetics, and some genetic indicators and have demonstrated the necessity of informed therapy choices, producing improved OS. However, current systems of stratification are limited to making generalizations based on population-wide data, with a substantial proportion of stratified patients who do not adhere to their assigned disease-progression cohort. Incorporating large-scale genomic data into these scoring systems will increase the granularity of features being assessed and enhance the complexity of the system to better model individual patients. Creating an enhanced risk-stratification model that leverages previously considered clinical and molecular features along with personal genomics is a substantive but important task that promises increased precision and therefore improved OS among MDS patients.

DISCLOSURE

The authors disclose no conflict of interest of this work.

REFERENCES

1. Vardiman JW, Thiele J, Arber DA, et al. The 2008 revision of the World Health Organization (WHO) classification of myeloid neoplasms and acute leukemia: Rationale and important changes. Blood 2009;114:937–51.
2. Tefferi A, Vardiman JW. Myelodysplastic syndromes: mechanisms of disease. Hematol Cell Ther 2009;38(5):363–80.
3. Fenaux P, Ades L. How we treat lower-risk myelodysplastic syndromes. Blood 2013;121(21):4280–6.
4. Greenberg PL, Stone RM, Al-Kali A, et al. Myelodysplastic syndromes, version 2.2017: clinical practice guidelines in oncology. J Natl Compr Canc Netw 2017; 15:60–87.
5. Malcovati L, Hellström-Lindberg E, Bowen D, et al. Diagnosis and treatment of primary myelodysplastic syndromes in adults: recommendations from the European LeukemiaNet. Blood 2013;122:2943–64.
6. Sekeres MA, Cutler C. How we treat higher-risk myelodysplastic syndromes. Blood 2014;123:829–36.

7. Garcia-Manero G, Shan J, Faderl S, et al. A prognostic score for patients with lower risk myelodysplastic syndrome. Leukemia 2008;22(3):538–43.

8. Greenberg P, Cox C, LeBeau MM, et al. International scoring system for evaluating prognosis in myelodysplastic syndromes. Blood 1997;89(6):2079–88. Available at: http://www.ncbi.nlm.nih.gov/pubmed/9058730.

9. Kantarjian H, O'Brien S, Ravandi F, et al. Proposal for a new risk model in myelodysplastic syndrome that accounts for events not considered in the original International Prognostic Scoring System. Cancer 2008;113(6):1351–61.

10. Pfeilstöcker M, Tuechler H, Sanz G, et al. Time-dependent changes in mortality and transformation risk in MDS. Blood 2016;128(7):902–10.

11. Haferlach T, Nagata Y, Grossmann V, et al. Landscape of genetic lesions in 944 patients with myelodysplastic syndromes. Leukemia 2014;28(2):241–7.

12. Nazha A, Narkhede M, Radivoyevitch T, et al. Incorporation of molecular data into the Revised International Prognostic Scoring System in treated patients with myelodysplastic syndromes. Leukemia 2016;30(11):2214–20.

13. Nazha Aziz, Sekeres MA, Komrokji R, et al. Validation of a post-hypomethylating agent failure prognostic model in myelodysplastic syndromes patients treated in a randomized controlled phase III trial of rigosertib vs. Best supportive care. Blood Cancer J 2017;7:644.

14. Greenberg PL, Attar E, Bennett JM, et al. Myelodysplastic syndromes: clinical practice guidelines in oncology. J Natl Compr Canc Netw 2013;11(7):838–74. Available at: http://www.ncbi.nlm.nih.gov/pubmed/23847220%0Ahttp://www.pubmedcentral.nih.gov/articlerender.fcgi?artid=PMC4000017.

15. Malcovati L, Germing U, Kuendgen A, et al. Time-dependent prognostic scoring system for predicting survival and leukemic evolution in myelodysplastic syndromes. J Clin Oncol 2007;25(23):3503–10.

16. Greenberg PL, Tuechler H, Schanz J, et al. Revised International Prognostic Scoring System for myelodysplastic syndromes. Blood 2012;120(12):2454–65.

17. Nazha Aziz, Seastone DP, Keng M, et al. The Revised International Prognostic Scoring System (IPSS-R) is not predictive of survival in patients with secondary myelodysplastic syndromes. Leuk Lymphoma 2015;56:3437–9.

18. Neukirchen J, Lauseker M, Blum S, et al. Validation of the Revised International Prognostic Scoring System (IPSS-R) in patients with myelodysplastic syndrome: a multicenter study. Leuk Res 2014;38(1):57–64.

19. Sekeres MA, Swern AS, Fenaux P, et al. Validation of the IPSS-R in lenalidomide-treated, lower-risk myelodysplastic syndrome patients with del(5q). Blood Cancer J 2014;4:e242.

20. Jabbour E, Garcia-Manero G, Batty N, et al. Outcome of patients with myelodysplastic syndrome after failure of decitabine therapy. Cancer 2010;116(16):3830–4.

21. Jabbour EJ, Garcia-Manero G, Strati P, et al. Outcome of patients with low-risk and intermediate-1-risk myelodysplastic syndrome after hypomethylating agent failure: a report on behalf of the MDS Clinical Research Consortium. Cancer 2015;121(6):876–82.

22. Prébet T, Gore SD, Esterni B, et al. Outcome of high-risk myelodysplastic syndrome after azacitidine treatment failure. J Clin Oncol 2011;29(24):3322–7.

23. Nazha Aziz, Komrokji RS, Garcia-Manero G, et al. The efficacy of current prognostic models in predicting outcome of patients with myelodysplastic syndromes at the time of hypomethylating agent failure. Haematologica 2016;101:e224–7.

24. Prebet T, Fenaux P, Vey N. Predicting outcome of patients with myelodysplastic syndromes after failure of azacitidine: validation of the North American MDS consortium scoring system. Haematologica 2016;101:e427–8.

25. Nazha A, Al-Issa K, Hamilton BK, et al. Adding molecular data to prognostic models can improve predictive power in treated patients with myelodysplastic syndromes. Leukemia 2017;31:2848–50.

26. Al-Issa K, Madanat YF, Mukherjee S, et al. Model heterogeneity in predicting outcomes of patients with myelodysplastic syndromes (MDS). Blood 2017; 130(Suppl 1):2972.

27. Papaemmanuil E, Gerstung M, Malcovati L, et al. Clinical and biological implications of driver mutations in myelodysplastic syndromes. Blood 2013;122(22): 3616–27.

28. Bejar R, Papaemmanuil E, Haferlach T, et al. Somatic mutations in MDS patients are associated with clinical features and predict prognosis independent of the IPSS-R: analysis of combined datasets from the international working group for prognosis in MDS-Molecular committee. Blood 2015;126(23).

29. Al-Issa K, Sekeres MA, Nielsen Ad, et al. TP53 mutations and outcome in patients with myelodysplastic syndromes (MDS). Blood 2016;128(22):4336.

30. Bejar R, Stevenson KE, Caughey B, et al. Somatic mutations predict poor outcome in patients with myelodysplastic syndrome after hematopoietic stem-cell transplantation. J Clin Oncol 2014;32(25):2691–8.

31. Della Porta MG, Gallì A, Bacigalupo A, et al. Clinical effects of driver somatic mutations on the outcomes of patients with myelodysplastic syndromes treated with allogeneic hematopoietic stem-cell transplantation. J Clin Oncol 2016;34(30): 3627–37.

32. Nazha Aziz, Komrokji RS, Meggendorfer M, et al. A personalized prediction model to risk stratify patients with myelodysplastic syndromes. Blood 2018; 132(Suppl 1):793. https://doi.org/10.1182/blood-2018-99-114774 (ASH Abstract). Available at:.

33. Yoshizato T, Nannya Y, Atsuta Y, et al. Impact of genetic alterations in stem-cell transplantation for myelodysplasia and secondary acute myeloid leukemia. Blood 2017;129(17):2347–58.

34. Lindsley RC, Saber W, Mar BG, et al. Prognostic mutations in myelodysplastic syndrome after stem-cell transplantation. N Engl J Med 2017;376(6):536–47.

Targeting Aberrant Splicing in Myelodysplastic Syndromes

Biologic Rationale and Clinical Opportunity

Andrew M. Brunner, MD[a,*], David P. Steensma, MD[b]

KEYWORDS

- RNA splicing • Alternative splicing • RNA splicing factors
- Myelodysplastic syndrome • Synthetic lethal mutations • Molecular targeted therapy

KEY POINTS

- Myelodysplastic syndromes (MDS) are enriched for somatic mutations in proteins involved in pre-mRNA splicing, specifically *SF3B1*, *SRSF2*, *U2AF1*, or *ZRSR2*.
- Alterations in pre-mRNA splicing in MDS may expose therapeutic vulnerabilities related to splicing itself or to effects caused by altered splicing in the cells.
- Identification of multiple targets in splicing factor mutated cells may lead to novel drugs or novel drug combinations for the treatment of MDS and other myeloid neoplasms in the future.

INTRODUCTION

Myelodysplastic syndromes (MDS) are cancers of the bone marrow with diverse clinical presentations, collectively characterized by clonally restricted hematopoiesis, cytopenias, dysplastic cell morphology, functional blood cell defects, and a risk of clonal evolution, including progression to acute leukemia.[1–3] Patients with MDS face complications related to or exacerbated by bone marrow failure and have a high symptom burden,[4,5] and higher-risk forms of MDS have a poor prognosis with a median survival measured ranging from months to a few years.[6,7] Treatment of lower-risk MDS often is focused on alleviating symptoms related to ineffective clonal hematopoiesis—most commonly centering on amelioration of anemia—whereas in higher-risk

Funding: Dr A.M. Brunner's work on this project was supported in part by the SPORE in Myeloid Malignancies career enhancement program (NCI 1P50CA206963). Dr D.P. Steensma is supported by the Edward P Evans Foundation, the James & Lois Champy Fund and NCI 1P50CA206963 SPORE.

[a] Massachusetts General Hospital, Zero Emerson Place, Suite 118, Boston, MA 02114, USA;
[b] Dana-Farber Cancer Institute, 450 Brookline Avenue, Boston, MA 02215, USA
* Corresponding author.
E-mail address: abrunner@mgh.harvard.edu

MDS, therapy usually is intended to alter the course of disease and prolong survival.[8] Currently, therapeutic options for MDS are limited, and no new therapies have been approved by regulatory authorities for MDS-related indications for approximately 15 years,[9] although that may change soon.

Although almost all patients with MDS have somatic mutations in hematopoietic cells (mostly in genes encoding epigenetic modifiers, spliceosome components, and transcription factors), to date, no available therapies are particularly specific for a given molecularly defined subset of MDS. For instance, although a majority of patients with MDS with del(5q) are likely to have improvements to their transfusion burden when treated with lenalidomide,[10] some do not, and conversely a smaller proportion of patients without del(5q) also may see improvement in transfusion needs and transfusion independence during lenalidomide therapy.[11,12] Similarly, the hypomethylating agents azacitidine and decitabine are routinely used as disease-modifying chemotherapeutics for patients with higher-risk disease, but mutation patterns have only modest effect on clinical response and such data are not used in practice for treatment decision making.[13(p2),14,15] New therapies that selectively target malignant clones while sparing healthy bone marrow (and ideally thus providing favorable toxicity profile) are desperately needed.

A challenge in developing new clinical therapeutics has been the limitations of preclinical in vivo models of MDS[16]—as a result, many therapeutics in MDS to date have been borrowed from acute myeloid leukemia (AML) or other hematological malignancies in which such models are better developed. This barrier to drug development has been changing thanks to a greater understanding of the genetic composition of MDS and novel mouse models that provide insight into MDS genetics.[17–19] Sequencing efforts have identified frequent recurrent mutations in MDS that allow for the identification of clonal origin and how disease evolves over time.[3,20–22] These efforts identified frequent, recurrent mutations in pre-mRNA splicing that appear to be early events in the development of MDS.[23–27] Splicing factor mutations are present in more than half of MDS and chronic myelomonocytic leukemia (CMML) cases and are associated with specific phenotypic findings, such as SF3B1 and ring sideroblasts,[28(p1),29(p1)] or SRSF2 enrichment in CMML.[30]

This review discusses the rationale for targeting pre-mRNA splicing in MDS, including preclinical insights into the effects of splicing factor mutations and how they may present therapeutic vulnerabilities, and early clinical data from studies in progress are summarized. The spliceosome is an appealing target due to the prevalence of splicing factor mutations in MDS, presence of mutations in early malignant progenitors, and potential for exploiting synthetic lethality strategies. Nonetheless, splicing is such a fundamental biological process that the therapeutic window of splicing modulation may be narrow, and much work is needed to understand how to target splicing and test novel therapeutic combinations in order to change the MDS treatment paradigm.

PRECLINICAL RATIONALE

Somatic mutations in pre-mRNA splicing factors are seen in several cancers, including solid tumors (notably uveal melanoma) and lymphoid malignancies, such as chronic lymphocytic leukemia.[27(p1),31–34(p1)] These mutations are enriched in myeloid neoplasms, specifically in MDS, CMML, and AML (especially secondary AML arising from MDS). In MDS, mutations in splicing factors occur most often in SF3B1, U2AF1, SRSF2, and less frequently ZRSR2.[25] Combined, splicing factor mutations represent the most frequently acquired recurrently mutated gene in MDS[35] and thus are of interest as possible therapeutic targets.[36]

Splicing factor mutations result in characteristics splicing alterations, which can then be measured as a biomarker.[37] Normal splicing proceeds through the identification of a 5′ splice site and 3′ splice site at either end of each intron to be spliced together as well as a branch point sequence upstream of the 3′ splice site and polypyrimidine tract that are critical for the identification of exons and splicing accuracy.[38] In the initial steps of mRNA splicing, the 5′ site is identified and bound to the branch point sequence by the U1 and U2 small nuclear ribonucleoproteins (snRNPs), the latter of which contains SF3B1, which binds to the branch point sequence. U2AF1 is involved in recognizing the 3′ splice site, whereas SRSF2, a member of the serine/arginine protein family, functions as a splicing enhancer, with a role in exon recognition. ZRSR2 appears to have a role analogous to U2AF1 but as part of the minor splicing complex. Mutations in these splicing factors result in characteristic alterations in pre-mRNA splicing based on these functions[39]: mutations in SF3B1 result in alternative branchpoint usage,[40,41] mutations in U2AF1 are associated with altered splice site recognition,[42] and mutations in SRSF2 result in altered recognition of exon splicing enhancers, inducing altered splicing of several proteins, including critical regulators of hematopoiesis.[43(p2)]

At the same time, splicing does not happen in a vacuum; rather, splicing is coupled with RNA transcription in a dynamic fashion.[44–46] This has the effect that any perturbations in splicing can cascade into the normal processing of mRNA, potentially slowing elongation. Alterations in RNA transcription may lead to increased RNA:DNA hybrid structures, termed R-loops,[47] which can effect DNA integrity and lead to single-strand breaks.[48,49] In response, ataxia telangiectasia and Rad3-related (ATR) signaling is activated, with eventual R-loop resolution.[50] The downstream effects of alternative splicing on such integral cellular functions as pre-mRNA transcription may profurther targets for therapeutic intervention in splicing factor mutated cells.

Mutual Exclusivity of Splicing Factor Mutations

Nearly all MDS cases can be characterized by at least 1 recurrent somatic mutation using a relatively small panel of approximately 100 myeloid genes of interest,[35,51–53] the most frequently mutated family of genes being those in the splicing apparatus.[51] These mutations almost always are mutually exclusive of one another,[26,31,54] meaning that (with rare exception) a patient sample harbors only 1 splicing mutation. Instances of more than 1 splicing factor mutation identified often may represent separate subclonal events. In addition, splicing factor mutations are heterozygous events, and the presence of the wild-type allele appears necessary for cell survival.[55] These factors suggest that mutations in the splicing apparatus, although frequent in MDS, nonetheless result in a state of dependence on some wild-type splicing function, with strong negative selection for homozygous mutations or mutations in multiple splicing factor genes in the same cell.

Splicing Factor Mutations as Early Clonal Events

Serial sequencing of MDS patient samples over time shows that dynamic clonal changes may occur and can be associated with changes in clinical and pathologic behavior.[56,57] Some mutations, including those commonly seen in secondary AML, such as FLT3, PTPN11, WT1, IDH1, NPM1, IDH2, and NRAS, are more commonly late events, occurring around the time of disease transformation.[57] This contrasts with splicing mutations, which usually are present early in the course of disease.[23(p1),58,59(p1)] Mutations in SF3B1, SRSF2, or U2AF1 tend to persist after treatment even when clinical response occurs,[58,60] further supporting the hypothesis that these mutations are present in an early progenitor and critical to the initial development of MDS. If these mutations are early in disease, it also suggests that therapies targeting splicing factor mutations may be more likely to have an impact on the malignant progenitor clone and perhaps thus more likely to elicit durable responses.

Preclinical Models of Splicing Factor Mutant Myelodysplastic Syndromes

Efforts to recapitulate genomically accurate murine models of myelodysplasia have led to new models for testing therapeutic combinations for treating MDS and greater insights into its pathogenesis (**Fig. 1**).[61–63] One such murine model utilized inducible SRSF2 P95H, a mutation hotspot in human MDS. In this murine model, the investigators showed that homozygous loss of *SRSF2* resulted in failed hematopoiesis, but conditional expression of P95H mutations in SRSF2 yielded a myeloid dysplasia phenotype.[43] Splicing factor mutations do not appear to result in loss of function (which may be lethal), but rather alter splicing preferences; in the SRSF2 murine model, disruption of SRSF2 function resulted in alternative splicing of several key hematopoietic regulators like *EZH2*. In a different inducible murine model of U2AF1 S34 F, heterozygosity for this mutation recapitulated an MDS phenotype and resulted in aberrant splicing involving genes recurrently mutated in MDS and AML, among others.[64] Curiously, these inducible models of splicing factor mutations can recapitulate some aspects of the MDS phenotype, but splicing mutant cells have a competitive

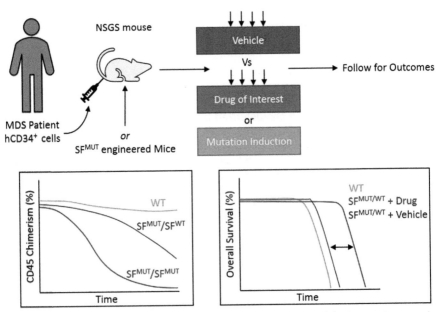

Fig. 1. General schema of splicing factor mutated MDS murine models. A prototype murine model of MDS. MDS progenitor cells may be introduced into mice through several methods, including using patient samples or engineering mice with inducible splicing factor mutations. After infusion/induction, these cells can be tested either comparing wild-type (WT) or mutant (SF^MUT) populations alone or in combination with a drug of interest (eg, spliceosome modulator or ATR inhibitor). Competitive transplantation studies show exhaustion of the clones harboring splicing factor mutations, that is, hastened in homozygous mutations. Spliceosome modulation appears to improve survival when administered to mice with splicing factor mutated leukemic xenografts. hCD34+, human CD34+; NSGS, NOD scid gamma SGM3.

disadvantage with wild-type cells in cotransplantation experiments, in contrast to what is seen in human MDS (see **Fig. 1**).

Synthetic Lethality in Splicing Factor Mutant Cells

A key question raised by the frequency of splicing factor mutations is whether and how these mutations could be targeted for therapeutic effect. Using murine models with mutated *SRSF2* or *U2AF1,* the effects of specific chemotherapies have been testing for signals of selective activity against mutant cells (see **Fig. 1**).[62,63] In 1 study, mice engineered to express the SRSF2 P95H mutation received the spliceosome modulator E7107, an SF3B1 inhibitor. In this model, there was no significant difference in survival between *SRSF2*[P95H/+] mice and *SRSF2*[WT] mice, but those mice with heterozygous SRSF2 P95H mutations who were exposed to E7107 had prolonged survival.[62] Similarly, in a study evaluating hematopoietic cells expressing *U2AF1*[S34F/+], exposure to sudemycin compounds, which bind to the SF3B1 protein in the spliceosome, attenuated expansion of *U2AF1*-mutated progenitor cells in a mouse transplant model.[63] These and other studies have led to a hypothesized mechanism of action for spliceosome modulators: there is a degree of tolerable splicing dysfunction within a cell, but further alteration of splicing results in a state where the cell can no longer compensate and leads to selective cell death (**Fig. 2**).

Interaction with Transcription and DNA Damage

Because splicing occurs in conjunction with mRNA transcription, alterations in splicing can affect the efficiency and integrity of transcription. As discussed previously, alternative splicing slows the replication fork and results in DNA:RNA hybrid

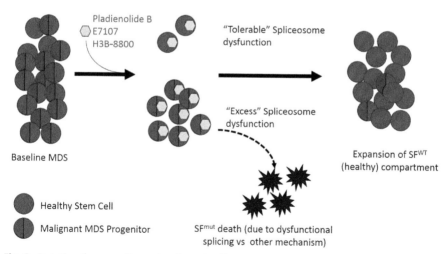

Fig. 2. Putative therapeutic mechanism of spliceosome modulator therapies in splicing factor mutated cells. At diagnosis, patients with MDS have largely malignant hematopoiesis arising from MDS progenitors; in splicing factor mutated MDS, normal splicing function is diminished and maintained by the wild-type allele. Modulators of the spliceosome are thought to further alter splicing; healthy progenitor cells are able to tolerate this modulation, whereas cells with a splicing factor mutation have excessive spliceosome dysfunction leading to cell death. This hypothetically results in the expansion of the healthy cell compartment and restoration of normal hematopoiesis. SF[mut], splicing factor mutant; SF[WT], splicing factor wild type.

structures, termed R-loops. R-loops are unstable structures that displace the non-hybridized DNA strand, resulting in single-stranded DNA, which activates a DNA damage response mediated through ATR signaling.[48,65,66] Interrupting this DNA damage response may hamper genomic integrity and lead to selective apoptosis of splicing factor mutant cells.[67–69] Alternatively, cumulative DNA damage as well as the buildup of alternatively spliced isoforms may yield tumor-enriched antigens that enhance immunogenicity on their own or in combination with immuno-oncologic therapies.[70,71]

CLINICAL STUDIES

Several therapies have recently entered clinical trials to test the preclinical rationale of targeting the spliceosome itself or associated pathways (**Table 1**). Although clinical results are preliminary, early signals from these studies are likely to greatly influence our understanding of spliceosome function in both wild-type and mutated cells, including the role of splicing factor mutations in MDS pathogenesis and treatment.

Modulating Spliceosome Function

Some of the first human studies to evaluate a spliceosome modulator investigated the compound E7107. Two phase 1 studies of E7107-enrolled patients with advanced solid tumors (NCT00459823 and NCT00499499).[72,73] Although no patients on these studies had a diagnosis of MDS, the toxicities encountered may be informative to spliceosome modulators in general. A total of 56 patients were enrolled between the 2 studies; the maximum tolerated dose of E7107 as an intravenous infusion was 4.3 mg/m^2 when given on days 1 and 8 of a 21-day cycle, or 4 mg/m^2 when dosed on days 1, 8, and 15 of a 28-day cycle. Dose-limiting toxicities across the 2 studies included gastrointestinal toxicity (diarrhea, vomiting, nausea, and abdominal cramping), anorexia, dehydration, and myocardial infarction. Also noted were 3 patients who experienced irreversible visual toxicity—1 with blurred vision and central scotomas and 2 others with vision loss; these events resulted in cessation of further study of this agent. Investigators did observe a dose-dependent change in mRNA splicing in cells from E7107-treated patients.[73]

Table 1			
Active clinical trials for splicing factor mutated myelodysplastic syndromes			
Drug	**Target**	**NCT Number**	**Notes**
H3B-8800	Small molecule modulator of SF3B1	NCT02841540	Dose escalation on 2 schedules: 5 d on, 9 d off, or 21 d of 28 d
GSK3326595	Reversible inhibitor of PRMT5	NCT03614728	Dose escalation followed by 3 parallel study expansion arms in monotherapy or in combination with azacitidine
JNJ-64619178	Inhibitor of PRMT5	NCT03573310	Dose escalation and tolerability, evaluating in lower-risk MDS
AZD6738	Small molecular ATR inhibitor	NCT03770429	Single-agent AZD6738 in higher-risk MDS, CMML, and lower-risk MDS

H3B-8800 is an orally bioavailable small molecule modulator of SF3B1 that shares a pladienolide chemical backbone but is molecularly distinct from E7107. Preclinical data confirmed selective cytotoxic activity against splicing factor mutated leukemia in xenograft models.[74] H3B-8800 has been studied in a phase 1 dose escalation trial enrolling patients with AML, MDS, and CMML, with preliminary data reported to date (NCT02841540).[75,76] A total of 81 patients were enrolled in dose escalation cohorts, evaluating doses of 1 mg to 40 mg administered either 5 days on/9 days off or on days 1 to 21 of a 28-day cycle. Dose-limiting toxicities included bone marrow failure in a patient with lower-risk MDS treated at 7 mg on the 5-days-on/9-days-off schedule and nausea and QTcF interval prolongation at 20 mg on the schedule of days 1 to 21 of 28. There was a dose-dependent increase in plasma levels of H3B-8800 as well as evidence of on-target alternative splicing in hematopoietic cells proportional to dose increases.[76] The drug generally was tolerable with several patients receiving treatment for over 2 years' duration.

Other spliceosome modulators are under development, including sudemycin D6,[77] Pladienolide-B, and FD-895, although none has yet been tested in human subjects[78]; there also is significant interest in novel combination therapies incorporating spliceosome modulation with other therapies in MDS.

Inhibition of Protein Arginine Methyltransferase 5

Protein arginine methyltransferase 5 (PRMT5) is essential to the formation of snRNPs and the spliceosome machinery. Inhibition of PRMT5 results in increased alternative splicing patterns[79] and also may impair homologous recombination DNA repair.[80] As such, PRMT5 is being explored as a target among tumors with spliceosome mutations.

GSK3326595 is a specific and reversible inhibitor of PRMT5 and has preclinical activity in several tumors; cell lines treated with GSK3326595 showed increased alternative splicing, and p53 activation due to alternative splicing of MDM4 was observed.[81] This compound has been studied in a phase 1 dose escalation study in solid tumors and non-Hodgkin lymphoma (NCT02783300)[82] and more recently is under investigation in myeloid neoplasms, including AML, MDS, and CMML (NCT03614728).

Another PRMT5 inhibitor in early human study is JNJ-64619178. This agent is orally bioavailable and shows preclinical efficacy in several tumors, including AML.[83] A study in patients with non-Hodgkin lymphoma and advanced solid tumors, as well as lower-risk MDS, is currently enrolling (NCT03573310).

Splicing-induced Immune Responses

Splicing factor mutations may result in generation of clonal cell-restricted neoantigens that can be recognized by the immune system.[71] Several studies are actively investigating the role of immunotherapy in MDS as monotherapy or in combination with hypomethylating agents, including the anti–CTLA-4 therapy ipilimumab and the anti–PD-1 or PD-L1 therapies nivolumab, pembrolizumab, and atezolizumab.[84,85] Although not specific to MDS harboring splicing factor mutations per se, analysis of mutation patterns and clinical responses in patients enrolled on these studies will be informative. Preliminary data suggest relatively low single-agent response rates to immune checkpoint inhibitors, restricted largely to arms containing CTLA-4 inhibition.[84] Moreover, several patients have experienced immune-related toxicities, including pulmonary complications, that need to be mitigated if these agents have a future in MDS.

DNA Damage Response

As noted, splicing factor mutations have effects on RNA transcription, resulting in the activation of a DNA damage response. Early data suggest that this occurs by recruitment of RPA to the area of R-loop formation, activating ATR signaling and the CHK1-Wee1 axis.[68] Inhibiting this DNA damage response may provide another target in splicing factor mutated as well as splicing wild-type MDS.

AZD6738 is an orally bioavailable selective inhibitor of ATR that has been studied in solid tumors as monotherapy and, because it may potentiate chemotherapy-induced DNA damage, paired with several other agents,[86(p67),87] including other DNA repair agents like poly(adenosine diphosphate-ribose) polymerase.[88] Mutations in the spliceosome result in constitutively increased R-loop formation and resultant ATR activation compared with wild-type cells.[68] Blunting the DNA damage response by inhibiting ATR results in synthetical lethal death preferentially in splicing factor mutated cells.[67] A clinical trial of AZD6738 in MDS and CMML currently is under way to test this hypothesis (NCT03770429). Other targets in this pathway, such as CHK1 and Wee1, may provide avenues for future study as well.

SUMMARY

The discovery of recurrent genetic mutations in MDS patient samples promises to bring an immense arsenal of targeted therapies to this extremely heterogeneous and treatment-refractory group of hematologic malignancies. A curious finding is the central, prominent role that mutations in the spliceosome machinery seem to play in this disease. These mutations occur early in the evolution of MDS and persist during treatment and over time. Splicing factor mutations are mutually exclusive of one another, and although each mutated splicing factor results in distinct and different downstream effects on splice isoforms, there are several common mis-spliced regulatory proteins. For all that has been discovered regarding splicing factor mutations in MDS, numerous questions remain, including how spliceosome mutations confer a clonal advantage and how best to exploit these mutations in the treatment of patients with this cancer. Nonetheless, the field is dynamic and evolving, with several currently enrolling trials targeting the pathways outlined in this review. Moreover, the identification of multiple potential targets against splicing factor mutations suggests the promise of novel:novel targeted combinations for patients with MDS, which may spare traditional chemotherapies altogether.

REFERENCES

1. Steensma DP. Myelodysplastic syndromes. Mayo Clin Proc 2015;90(7):969–83.
2. Brunner AM, Steensma DP. Recent advances in the cellular and molecular understanding of myelodysplastic syndromes: implications for new therapeutic approaches. Clin Adv Hematol Oncol 2018;16(1):56–66.
3. da Silva-Coelho P, Kroeze LI, Yoshida K, et al. Clonal evolution in myelodysplastic syndromes. Nat Commun 2017;8:15099.
4. Brunner AM, Blonquist TM, Hobbs GS, et al. Risk and timing of cardiovascular death among patients with myelodysplastic syndromes. Blood Adv 2017;1(23): 2032–40.
5. Steensma DP. Graphical representation of clinical outcomes for patients with myelodysplastic syndromes. Leuk Lymphoma 2016;57(1):17–20.
6. Greenberg P, Cox C, LeBeau MM, et al. International scoring system for evaluating prognosis in myelodysplastic syndromes. Blood 1997;89(6):2079–88.

7. Greenberg PL, Tuechler H, Schanz J, et al. Revised international prognostic scoring system for myelodysplastic syndromes. Blood 2012;120(12):2454–65.

8. Steensma DP. Myelodysplastic syndromes current treatment algorithm 2018. Blood Cancer J 2018;8(5):47.

9. Sekeres MA, Steensma DP. Boulevard of broken dreams: drug approval for older adults with acute myeloid leukemia. J Clin Oncol 2012;30(33):4061–3.

10. List A, Dewald G, Bennett J, et al. Lenalidomide in the myelodysplastic syndrome with chromosome 5q deletion. N Engl J Med 2006;355(14):1456–65.

11. Raza A, Reeves JA, Feldman EJ, et al. Phase 2 study of lenalidomide in transfusion-dependent, low-risk, and intermediate-1-risk myelodysplastic syndromes with karyotypes other than deletion 5q. Blood 2008;111(1):86–93.

12. Toma A, Kosmider O, Chevret S, et al. Lenalidomide with or without erythropoietin in transfusion-dependent erythropoiesis-stimulating agent-refractory lower-risk MDS without 5q deletion. 2016. Available at: https://hal-univ-rennes1.archives-ouvertes.fr/hal-01321412. Accessed July 15, 2019.

13. Itzykson R, Kosmider O, Cluzeau T, et al. Impact of TET2 mutations on response rate to azacitidine in myelodysplastic syndromes and low blast count acute myeloid leukemias. Leukemia 2011;25(7):1147–52.

14. Bejar R, Lord A, Stevenson K, et al. TET2 mutations predict response to hypomethylating agents in myelodysplastic syndrome patients. Blood 2014;124(17): 2705–12.

15. Schroeder MA, DeZern AE. Do somatic mutations in de novo MDS predict for response to treatment? Hematology 2015;2015(1):317–28.

16. Beurlet S, Chomienne C, Padua RA. Engineering mouse models with myelodysplastic syndrome human candidate genes; how relevant are they? Haematologica 2013;98(1):10–22.

17. Zhou T, Kinney MC, Scott LM, et al. Revisiting the case for genetically engineered mouse models in human myelodysplastic syndrome research. Blood 2015; 126(9):1057–68.

18. Song Y, Rongvaux A, Taylor A, et al. A highly efficient and faithful MDS patient-derived xenotransplantation model for pre-clinical studies. Nat Commun 2019; 10. https://doi.org/10.1038/s41467-018-08166-x.

19. Suragani RNVS, Cadena SM, Cawley SM, et al. Transforming growth factor-β superfamily ligand trap ACE-536 corrects anemia by promoting late-stage erythropoiesis. Nat Med 2014;20(4):408–14.

20. Hsu J, Reilly A, Hayes BJ, et al. Reprogramming identifies functionally distinct stages of clonal evolution in myelodysplastic syndromes. Blood 2019;134(2): 186–98.

21. Polgarova K, Vargova K, Kulvait V, et al. Somatic mutation dynamics in MDS patients treated with azacitidine indicate clonal selection in patients-responders. Oncotarget 2017;8(67):111966–78.

22. Uy GL, Duncavage EJ, Chang GS, et al. Dynamic changes in the clonal structure of MDS and AML in response to epigenetic therapy. Blood 2015;126(23):610.

23. Graubert TA, Shen D, Ding L, et al. Recurrent mutations in the U2AF1 splicing factor in myelodysplastic syndromes. Nat Genet 2012;44(1):53–7.

24. Makishima H, Visconte V, Sakaguchi H, et al. Mutations in the spliceosome machinery, a novel and ubiquitous pathway in leukemogenesis. Blood 2012; 119(14):3203–10.

25. Saez B, Walter MJ, Graubert TA. Splicing factor gene mutations in hematologic malignancies. Blood 2017;129(10):1260–9.

26. Yoshida K, Sanada M, Shiraishi Y, et al. Frequent pathway mutations of splicing machinery in myelodysplasia. Nature 2011;478(7367):64–9.

27. Quesada V, Conde L, Villamor N, et al. Exome sequencing identifies recurrent mutations of the splicing factor SF3B1 gene in chronic lymphocytic leukemia. Nat Genet 2012;44(1):47.

28. Malcovati L, Karimi M, Papaemmanuil E, et al. SF3B1 mutation identifies a distinct subset of myelodysplastic syndrome with ring sideroblasts. Blood 2015;126(2): 233–41.

29. Papaemmanuil E, Cazzola M, Boultwood J, et al. Somatic SF3B1 mutation in mye-lodysplasia with ring sideroblasts. N Engl J Med 2011;365(15):1384–95.

30. Meggendorfer M, Roller A, Haferlach T, et al. SRSF2 mutations in 275 cases with chronic myelomonocytic leukemia (CMML). Blood 2012;120(15):3080–8.

31. Seiler M, Peng S, Agrawal AA, et al. Somatic mutational landscape of splicing factor genes and their functional consequences across 33 cancer types. Cell Rep 2018;23(1):282–96.e4.

32. Scott LM, Rebel VI. Acquired mutations that affect Pre-mRNA splicing in hemato-logic malignancies and solid tumors. J Natl Cancer Inst 2013;105(20):1540–9.

33. Bejar R. Splicing factor mutations in cancer. Adv Exp Med Biol 2016;907:215–28.

34. Martin M, Maßhöfer L, Temming P, et al. Exome sequencing identifies recurrent somatic mutations in EIF1AX and SF3B1 in uveal melanoma with disomy 3. Nat Genet 2013;45(8):933.

35. Papaemmanuil E, Gerstung M, Malcovati L, et al. Clinical and biological implica-tions of driver mutations in myelodysplastic syndromes. Blood 2013;122(22): 3616–27.

36. Lee SC-W, Abdel-Wahab O. Therapeutic targeting of splicing in cancer. Nat Med 2016;22(9):976–86.

37. Pellagatti A, Armstrong RN, Steeples V, et al. Impact of spliceosome mutations on RNA splicing in myelodysplasia: dysregulated genes/pathways and clinical asso-ciations. Blood 2018;132(12):1225–40.

38. Yoshimi A, Abdel-Wahab O. Molecular pathways: understanding and targeting mutant spliceosomal proteins. Clin Cancer Res 2017;23(2):336–41.

39. Shiozawa Y, Malcovati L, Gallì A, et al. Aberrant splicing and defective mRNA production induced by somatic spliceosome mutations in myelodysplasia. Nat Commun 2018;9(1):3649.

40. Alsafadi S, Houy A, Battistella A, et al. Cancer-associated SF3B1 mutations affect alternative splicing by promoting alternative branchpoint usage. Nat Commun 2016;7:10615.

41. Darman RB, Seiler M, Agrawal AA, et al. Cancer-associated SF3B1 hotspot mu-tations induce Cryptic 3' splice site selection through use of a different branch point. Cell Rep 2015;13(5):1033–45.

42. Ilagan JO, Ramakrishnan A, Hayes B, et al. U2AF1 mutations alter splice site recognition in hematological malignancies. Genome Res 2015;25(1):14–26.

43. Kim E, Ilagan JO, Liang Y, et al. SRSF2 mutations contribute to myelodysplasia by mutant-specific effects on exon recognition. Cancer Cell 2015;27(5):617–30.

44. Schor IE, Gómez Acuña LI, Kornblihtt AR. Coupling between transcription and alternative splicing. Cancer Treat Res 2013;158:1–24.

45. Montes M, Becerra S, Sánchez-Álvarez M, et al. Functional coupling of transcrip-tion and splicing. Gene 2012;501(2):104–17.

46. Bentley DL. Coupling mRNA processing with transcription in time and space. Nat Rev Genet 2014;15(3):163–75.

47. Hamperl S, Cimprich KA. The contribution of co-transcriptional RNA:DNA hybrid structures to DNA damage and genome instability. DNA Repair (Amst) 2014;19: 84–94.

48. Crossley MP, Bocek M, Cimprich KA. R-Loops as cellular regulators and genomic threats. Mol Cell 2019;73(3):398–411.

49. Aguilera A, Gómez-González B. Genome instability: a mechanistic view of its causes and consequences. Nat Rev Genet 2008;9(3):204–17.

50. Cimprich KA, Cortez D. ATR: an essential regulator of genome integrity. Nat Rev Mol Cell Biol 2008;9(8):616–27.

51. Haferlach T, Nagata Y, Grossmann V, et al. Landscape of genetic lesions in 944 patients with myelodysplastic syndromes. Leukemia 2014;28(2):241–7.

52. Lindsley RC. Uncoding the genetic heterogeneity of myelodysplastic syndrome. Hematology 2017;2017(1):447–52.

53. Thol F, Kade S, Schlarmann C, et al. Frequency and prognostic impact of mutations in SRSF2, U2AF1, and ZRSR2 in patients with myelodysplastic syndromes. Blood 2012;119(15):3578–84.

54. Yoshida K, Ogawa S. Splicing factor mutations and cancer. Wiley Interdiscip Rev RNA 2014;5(4):445–59.

55. Fei DL, Motowski H, Chatrikhi R, et al. Wild-type U2AF1 antagonizes the splicing program characteristic of U2AF1-mutant tumors and is required for cell survival. PLoS Genet 2016;12(10):e1006384.

56. Steensma DP, Bejar R, Jaiswal S, et al. Clonal hematopoiesis of indeterminate potential and its distinction from myelodysplastic syndromes. Blood 2015; 126(1):9–16.

57. Makishima H, Yoshizato T, Yoshida K, et al. Dynamics of clonal evolution in myelodysplastic syndromes. Nat Genet 2017;49(2):204–12.

58. Mossner M, Jann J-C, Wittig J, et al. Mutational hierarchies in myelodysplastic syndromes dynamically adapt and evolve upon therapy response and failure. Blood 2016;128(9):1246–59.

59. Mian SA, Rouault-Pierre K, Smith AE, et al. SF3B1 mutant MDS-initiating cells may arise from the haematopoietic stem cell compartment. Nat Commun 2015;6: 10004.

60. Wu S-J, Kuo Y-Y, Hou H-A, et al. The clinical implication of SRSF2 mutation in patients with myelodysplastic syndrome and its stability during disease evolution. Blood 2012;120(15):3106–11.

61. Mupo A, Seiler M, Sathiaseelan V, et al. Hemopoietic-specific *Sf3b1*-K700E knock-in mice display the splicing defect seen in human MDS but develop anemia without ring sideroblasts. Leukemia 2017;31(3):720–7.

62. Lee SC-W, Dvinge H, Kim E, et al. Modulation of splicing catalysis for therapeutic targeting of leukemias with spliceosomal mutations. Nat Med 2016;22(6):672–8.

63. Shirai CL, White BS, Tripathi M, et al. Mutant U2AF1-expressing cells are sensitive to pharmacological modulation of the spliceosome. Nat Commun 2017;8:14060.

64. Shirai CL, Ley JN, White BS, et al. Mutant U2AF1 expression alters hematopoiesis and Pre-mRNA splicing in vivo. Cancer Cell 2015;27(5):631–43.

65. Chen L, Chen J-Y, Huang Y-J, et al. The augmented R-Loop is a unifying mechanism for myelodysplastic syndromes induced by high-risk splicing factor mutations. Mol Cell 2018;69(3):412–25.e6.

66. Flynn RL, Zou L. ATR: a master conductor of cellular responses to DNA replication stress. Trends Biochem Sci 2011;36(3):133–40.

67. Nguyen HD, Leong WY, Li W, et al. Spliceosome mutations induce R Loop-associated sensitivity to ATR inhibition in myelodysplastic syndromes. Cancer Res 2018;78(18):5363–74.
68. Nguyen HD, Yadav T, Giri S, et al. Functions of replication Protein A as a sensor of R loops and a regulator of RNaseH1. Mol Cell 2017;65(5):832–47.e4.
69. Nguyen HD, Zou L, Graubert TA. Targeting R-loop-associated ATR response in myelodysplastic syndrome. Oncotarget 2019;10(27):2581–2.
70. Kahles A, Lehmann K-V, Toussaint NC, et al. Comprehensive analysis of alternative splicing across tumors from 8,705 patients. Cancer Cell 2018;34(2):211–24.e6.
71. Hoyos LE, Abdel-Wahab O. Cancer-specific splicing changes and the potential for splicing-derived neoantigens. Cancer Cell 2018;34(2):181–3.
72. Hong DS, Kurzrock R, Naing A, et al. A phase I, open-label, single-arm, dose-escalation study of E7107, a precursor messenger ribonucleic acid (pre-mRNA) spliceosome inhibitor administered intravenously on days 1 and 8 every 21 days to patients with solid tumors. Invest New Drugs 2014;32(3):436–44.
73. Eskens FALM, Ramos FJ, Burger H, et al. Phase I pharmacokinetic and pharmacodynamic study of the first-in-class spliceosome inhibitor E7107 in patients with advanced solid tumors. Clin Cancer Res 2013;19(22):6296–304.
74. Seiler M, Yoshimi A, Darman R, et al. H3B-8800, an orally available small-molecule splicing modulator, induces lethality in spliceosome-mutant cancers. Nat Med 2018;24(4):497–504.
75. Steensma DP, Maris MB, Yang J, et al. H3B-8800-G0001-101: a first in human phase I study of a splicing modulator in patients with advanced myeloid malignancies. J Clin Oncol 2017;35(15_suppl):TPS7075.
76. Steensma D, Klimek V, Yang J, et al. Phase I dose escalation clinical trial of H3B-8800, a splicing modulator, in patients with advanced myeloid malignancies. EHA Library 2019;266651:PS1034.
77. Shi Y, Joyner AS, Shadrick W, et al. Pharmacodynamic assays to facilitate preclinical and clinical development of pre-mRNA splicing modulatory drug candidates. Pharmacol Res Perspect 2015;3(4). https://doi.org/10.1002/prp2.158.
78. Kashyap MK, Kumar D, Villa R, et al. Targeting the spliceosome in chronic lymphocytic leukemia with the macrolides FD-895 and pladienolide-B. Haematologica 2015;100(7):945–54.
79. Bezzi M, Teo SX, Muller J, et al. Regulation of constitutive and alternative splicing by PRMT5 reveals a role for Mdm4 pre-mRNA in sensing defects in the spliceosomal machinery. Genes Dev 2013;27(17):1903–16.
80. Hamard P-J, Santiago GE, Liu F, et al. PRMT5 regulates DNA repair by controlling the alternative splicing of histone-modifying enzymes. Cell Rep 2018;24(10):2643–57.
81. Gerhart SV, Kellner WA, Thompson C, et al. Activation of the p53-MDM4 regulatory axis defines the anti-tumour response to PRMT5 inhibition through its role in regulating cellular splicing. Sci Rep 2018;8. https://doi.org/10.1038/s41598-018-28002-y.
82. Rasco D, Tolcher A, Siu LL, et al. Abstract CT038: a phase I, open-label, dose-escalation study to investigate the safety, pharmacokinetics, pharmacodynamics, and clinical activity of GSK3326595 in subjects with solid tumors and non-Hodgkin's lymphoma. Cancer Res 2017;77(13 Supplement):CT038.
83. Millar HJ, Brehmer D, Verhulst T, et al. Abstract 950: in vivo efficacy and pharmacodynamic modulation of JNJ-64619178, a selective PRMT5 inhibitor, in human lung and hematologic preclinical models. Cancer Res 2019;79(13 Supplement):950.

84. Garcia-Manero G, Daver NG, Montalban-Bravo G, et al. A phase II study evaluating the combination of Nivolumab (Nivo) or Ipilimumab (Ipi) with azacitidine in Pts with previously treated or untreated Myelodysplastic Syndromes (MDS). Blood 2016;128(22):344.

85. Gerds AT, Scott BL, Greenberg PL, et al. PD-L1 blockade with atezolizumab in higher-risk myelodysplastic syndrome: an initial safety and efficacy analysis. Blood 2018;132(Suppl 1):466.

86. Dillon MT, Boylan Z, Smith D, et al. PATRIOT: a phase I study to assess the tolerability, safety and biological effects of a specific ataxia telangiectasia and Rad3-related (ATR) inhibitor (AZD6738) as a single agent and in combination with palliative radiation therapy in patients with solid tumours. Clin Transl Radiat Oncol 2018;12:16–20.

87. Foote KM, Nissink JWM, McGuire T, et al. Discovery and characterization of AZD6738, a potent inhibitor of ataxia telangiectasia mutated and Rad3 related (ATR) kinase with application as an anticancer agent. J Med Chem 2018;61(22):9889–907.

88. Lloyd R, Falenta K, Wijnhoven PW, et al. Abstract 337: The PARP inhibitor olaparib is synergistic with the ATR inhibitor AZD6738 in ATM deficient cancer cells. Cancer Res 2018;78(13 Supplement):337.

Luspatercept in Myelodysplastic Syndromes
Who and When?

Rami S. Komrokji, MD

KEYWORDS

• Myelodysplastic syndromes • Luspatercept • Anemia • Ineffective erythropoiesis

KEY POINTS

- Myelodysplastic syndromes (MDS) are characterized by ineffective erythropoiesis, which involves impaired early erythropoiesis as well as terminal erythroid differentiation.
- Impaired terminal erythroid maturation in MDS is transforming growth factor beta pathway mediated. The pathway is overactivated in patients with MDS, and ligands such as growth differentiation factor 11 are overexpressed.
- Luspatercept is an activin receptor type IIB fusion ligand trap novel agent. It neutralizes the ligands before binding the receptor and thus inhibits signaling through the receptor.
- Luspatercept showed promising activity for treating anemia in lower-risk patients with MDS with ring sideroblast subtypes.
- The MEDALIST phase 3 randomized double-blind placebo-controlled clinical trial showed higher rates of durable red blood cell transfusion independence with luspatercept, as well as hematological improvement, and was generally well tolerated.

INTRODUCTION

Anemia is the hallmark of myelodysplastic syndromes (MDS), a group of neoplastic stem cell diseases characterized clinically by bone marrow failure and the tendency to progress to acute myeloid leukemia (AML). MDS is one of the most common causes of anemia in elderly, and most patients with MDS become red blood cell (RBC) transfusion dependent (TD) during the course of their disease.[1,2] Anemia burden in MDS includes symptoms, exacerbating comorbidities affecting patients' quality of life, and the sequela of iron overload, as well as other complications of RBC-TD, as well as the costs encountered, which are substantial. Anemia and RBC-TD correlate with inferior outcomes in MDS.[3,4]

Treatment of anemia in lower-risk MDS (LR-MDS) is the main goal and remains an unmet challenge with few options currently available.[2] Erythroid-stimulating agents (ESAs) often represent the first step of management, with overall response rates of

Malignant Hematology Department, Moffitt Cancer Center and Research Institute, 12902 Magnolia Drive, Tampa, FL 33612, USA
E-mail address: rami.komrokji@moffitt.org

Hematol Oncol Clin N Am 34 (2020) 393–400
https://doi.org/10.1016/j.hoc.2019.10.004
0889-8588/20/© 2019 Elsevier Inc. All rights reserved.

20% to 40% and an 18-month to 24-month duration of response.[5] Lenalidomide is the standard of care for patients with deletion 5q MDS, in which 67% of patients become RBC transfusion independent (TI) with a 3-year median duration of response.[6] However, in non–deletion 5q MDS lenalidomide RBC-TI rates are 25% with less than a 1-year median duration of response.[7] Hypomethylating agents (HMAs) are used for treatment of anemia in LR-MDS, with 20% to 40% response rates reported.[8] In addition, immunosuppressive therapy is recommended only for a small subset of young patients with MDS who are not heavily RBC-TD.[9]

Recently, the role of the transforming growth factor beta (TGF-B) pathway in regulating erythropoiesis and its overactivation in patients with MDS has become more evident.[10] Targeting the TGF-B pathway is an appealing approach to improving anemia in LR-MDS. Novel fusion trap proteins neutralizing TGF-B ligands were explored in clinical trials. These proteins showed promising activity and reasonable safety, which it is hoped will lead to luspatercept being the next drug approved for the treatment of anemia in LR-MDS.[11]

INEFFECTIVE ERYTHROPOIESIS IN MYELODYSPLASTIC SYNDROMES

Normal erythropoiesis includes the early stage of hematopoietic stem cell proliferation and differentiation into erythroid progenitors and a later stage of terminal erythroid maturation into enucleated RBCs.[12] Ineffective erythropoiesis is the hallmark of MDS, evident morphologically by erythroid dysplasia. The defects include intrinsic clonal disease features as well as microenvironment inflammatory milieu, both of which contribute to impaired erythropoiesis in both early-stage and terminal erythroid differentiation.[12,13] Recently, it was shown that activation of the inflammasome, whether driven by genetic mutations or inflammatory signaling, forms a platform for accelerated pyroptotic cell death.[14] Impaired terminal erythroid differentiation in MDS through reduced levels of GATA-1 master regulator and TGF-B pathway ligands, such as growth differentiation factor 11 (GDF-11), which acts as a negative regulator for this step, became more apparent.[12]

TRANSFORMING GROWTH FACTOR BETA PATHWAY AND MYELODYSPLASTIC SYNDROME

The TGF-B receptors are a superfamily of serine/threonine kinase receptors. TGF-B superfamily receptors are grouped into 3 types: type I, type II, and type III. The TGF-B signaling pathway involves ligand binding to type II receptors, which recruits and phosphorylates type I receptors. Activin type II A and B receptors are members of the type II family receptors. The TGF-B receptor ligands are polypeptide growth factors, including TGF-B, activins, bone morphogenetic proteins, and GDF-11. These cytokines regulate several cellular processes during development, including hematopoiesis in adults.[15] Activin and GDF-11 have inhibitory effects on terminal erythropoiesis, distinct from the erythropoietin (epo) early regulatory role.[12] Following ligand binding and receptor phosphorylation, the SMAD signaling pathway becomes activated, including SMAD-2 and SMAD-4. SMAD-6 and SMAD-7 serve as regulatory inhibitory proteins.[15]

Impaired terminal erythroid maturation in MDS is TGF-B pathway mediated. SMAD-2 downstream mediators are overexpressed in MDS CD34+ cells. The increased TGF-B signaling in patients with MDS is related to decrease expression of the negative pathway regulator SMAD-7, which is reduced as result of microRNA-21 overexpression in patients with MDS. GDF-11 levels, a negative regulator of terminal erythrocyte differentiation, are increased in patients with MDS.[16–18]

LUSPATERCEPT A NOVEL AGENT TARGETING THE TRANSFORMING GROWTH FACTOR BETA PATHWAY

Luspatercept (ACE-536) is an activin receptor type IIB (ActRIIB) fusion ligand trap novel agent. The molecule consists of the extracellular domain of the TGF-B receptor linked to the human immunoglobulin (Ig) G_1 Fc domain. Luspatercept neutralizes the ligands before binding the receptor and thus inhibits signaling through the receptor.[11]

The murine analogue of luspatercept RAP-536 showed a robust increase in erythrocyte numbers and reduced or prevented anemia in mice models. Cotreatment with ACE-536 and epo produced a synergistic response. ACE-536 bound GDF11 and potently inhibited its mediated SMAD-2/3 signaling.[19] In humans, the first study included 34 postmenopausal female healthy volunteers. The dose was escalated until a dose-dependent increase in hemoglobin (Hgb) concentration was observed, beginning 7 days after initiation of treatment and maintained for several weeks following treatment.[20]

LUSPATERCEPT CLINICAL TRIALS

In a phase II multicenter dose-finding study with long-term extension, luspatercept was tested in patients with LR-MDS.[21] The PACE-MDS study enrolled low-risk and intermediate-risk International Prognostic Scoring System (IPSS) patients with MDS and nonproliferative chronic myelomonocytic leukemia with anemia regardless of RBC transfusion need. Patients were stratified as low transfusion burden (LTB; <4 RBC units transfused within 56 days before enrollment) or high transfusion burden (HTB; ≥4 RBC units within 56 days). Luspatercept was given subcutaneously every 3 weeks with doses ranging from 0.125 to 1.75 mg/kg for 5 doses in the escalation/expansion phase and up to 5 years in the extension study. The primary end point was erythroid hematological improvement (HI-E) by international working group (IWG) criteria 2006. Fifty-eight patients were enrolled, 27 in the escalation phase (0.125–1.75 mg/kg), 31 in the expansion phase (1–1.75 mg/kg), and 32 patients entered the extension study. The later part of the study was enriched with MDS ring sideroblasts (RS) subtypes. Of the 58 patients in the base study, 19 had low LTB and 39 had HTB. Of the 32 patients in the extension study, 13 had LTB and 19 had HTB.[21]

Overall, 32 of 51 patients (63%) receiving higher-dose luspatercept concentrations (0.75–1.75 mg/kg) achieved HI-E versus 2 of 9 patients (22%) receiving lower dose concentrations (0.125–0.5 mg/kg). Among the LTB patients treated with higher dose luspatercept, 11 out of 17 patients (65%) achieved HI-E, and 6 out of 8 patients who were requiring RBC transfusion became TI. Among the HTB patients treated with higher-dose luspatercept, 21 out 34 patients (62%) achieved HI-E, including 29% RBC-TI.[21]

There were no differences in response noted based on prior ESA use or lenalidomide use. Higher response rates were observed among patients with lower endogenous serum epo level. Among patients treated with higher dose concentrations of luspatercept, 29 of 42 patients with RS (69%) achieved HI-E versus 3 (43%) of 7 with no RS. The PACE study revealed promising activity and acceptable safety to conduct a randomized phase III clinical study.[21]

The MEDALIST was a phase III randomized, double-blind, placebo-controlled clinical trial of luspatercept to treat patients with very low, low, and intermediate IPSS-Revised (IPSS-R) MDS with ring sideroblasts and TD anemia.[22] The eligibility criteria included confirmed diagnosis of MDS with RS greater than or equal to 15% or greater than or equal to 5% and SF3B1 gene mutation, less than 5% myeloblasts on bone marrow, non–deletion 5q MDS, ESA failure, refractory or intolerant or if

ESA naive with serum epo level greater than 200 U/L, and no prior HMA or lenalidomide were allowed. Transfusion dependency was defined as requiring at least 2 U/8 wk and patients stratified as LTB and HTB as defined in the PACE study. Patients were 2:1 randomized between luspatercept 1 mg/kg subcutaneously every 21 days and placebo (dose escalation to 1.33 and 1.75 mg/kg allowed). The primary end point was RBC-TI greater than or equal to 8 weeks (weeks 1–24). The secondary end points were RBC-TI greater than or equal to 12 weeks (weeks 1–24 and weeks 24–48), HI-E by IWG 2006, and duration of response.[22]

The MEDALIST study randomized 153 patients to luspatercept and 76 patients to placebo, and there was no difference in baseline characteristics between the 2 groups. More than 90% of patients were refractory cytopenia with multilineage dysplasia and ring sideroblast (RCMD-RS) subtype, approximately 43% had greater than or equal to 6 units/8 wk RBC transfusion burden, less than 20% were intermediate-risk IPSS-R, 42% on luspatercept arm and 34% on placebo had endogenous serum epo level greater than or equal to 200 U/L, and most of the patients harbored SF3B1 mutation as expected. At the time of data presentation at the American Society of Hematology meeting, 46% and 8% of patients were remaining on treatment in the luspatercept arm and placebo, respectively.[22]

The rate of RBC transfusion independence for greater than or equal to 8 weeks (weeks 1–24) was 37.9% on luspatercept compared with 13.2% on placebo (P<.0001). The RBC-TI rate greater than or equal to 12 weeks (weeks 1–24) was 28.1% and 7.9%, respectively (P = .002), and for 1 to 48 weeks was 33% and 12%, respectively (P = .003). Approximately 40% of responders on luspatercept remained RBC-TI at 1 year. There was no difference in response rate to luspatercept based on baseline endogenous serum epo levels. The rate of reduction of greater than or equal to 4 U (weeks 1–24) was 48.6% compared with 14.3% for luspatercept and placebo, respectively (P<.0001). In patients with baseline transfusion burden less than 4 U/8 wk, the rate of Hgb increase of greater than or equal to 1.5 g/dL (weeks 1–24) was 63% with luspatercept compared with 5% with placebo (P<.0001).[22]

The most common adverse events were fatigue, diarrhea, nausea, asthenia, dizziness, and back pain. Adverse events leading to discontinuation of treatment were reported in 8.5% with luspatercept and 7.9% with placebo. AML progression was reported in 3 out of 153 patients (2%) in the luspatercept arm and 1 out of 76 patients (1.3%) in the placebo arm.[22] **Table 1** summarizes key findings from the PACE and MEDALIST studies.

LUSPATERCEPT: WHO AND WHEN?

The anticipated US Food and Drug Administration (FDA) approval based on the MEDALIST study will be for lower-risk patients with MDS with RS who are RBC-TD with a low chance of response, refractory or intolerant to ESA. The study defined RBC-TD as the need for at least 2 U/8 wk. The treatment would fill an unmet need for patients with MDS with RS after lenalidomide and HMA failure. The MEDALIST study excluded these patients; however, in the PACE study, which was highly enriched with RS subtype patients, 63% (5 out of 8 patients) with prior lenalidomide had HI-E reported.[22] The PACE and MEDALIST trials did not include patients after HMA failure.[21,22] Sotatercept, a novel fusion ligand trap agent against ActRIIB, was tested in a phase II multicenter dose-finding study in lower-risk patients with MDS for treatment of TD anemia.[23] Of 74 patients treated with sotatercept, 36 (49%) achieved HI-E and 20 (27%) achieved RBC transfusion independence. Thirty patients out of 51 (59%) with greater than or equal to 15% RSs achieved HI-E, and 4 patients

Table 1
Key findings from MEDALIST and PACE luspatercept myelodysplastic syndrome studies

Study	MEDALIST		PACE (0.75–1.75 mg/kg Dose)
Number of Patients	Luspatercept (153)	Placebo (76)	49
Baseline Characteristics			
Median Age (y)	71	72	71
WHO Subtype: RCMD-RS (%)	95	97	51
RBC Transfusion >4 Units/8 wk (%)	70	74	65
Intermediate-risk IPSS-R (%)	16	17	39
SF3B1 Mutation (%)	92	86	61
Serum Epo >200 U/L (%)	42	34	22
Prior Lenalidomide Exposure (%)	0	0	16
Efficacy Response (%)			
RBC-TI			
RBC-TI>8 wk (N)	38	13	38
RBC-TI in LTB Patients (N)	80	40	75
RBC-TI in Patients with Epo >200 U/L (N)	40	7	44
HI-E (N)	53	12	63
Median Duration of Response (wk)	31	14	60
AEs			
Fatigue (%)	27	13	7
Diarrhea (%)	22	9	5
Asthenia (%)	20	12	NR
Nausea (%)	20	8	2
Dizziness (%)	20	5	NR
Back Pain/Bone Pain (%)	19	7	12
Cough (%)	18	13	NR
Peripheral Edema (%)	16	17	2
Headache (%)	16	6	3
Dyspnea (%)	15	7	NR
Bronchitis (%)	11	1	NR
Constipation (%)	11	9	NR
Urinary Tract Infection (%)	11	5	NR
Fall (%)	10	12	NR
Treatment Discontinuation Because of AE (%)	9	8	3
AML/Increased Myeloblasts (%)	2	1	2

Reported different between MEDALIST and PACE including back pain, bone pain, leg pain, and arthralgia.

Abbreviations: AE, adverse event; NR, not reported; WHO, World Health Organization.

out of 18 (22%) with RSs less than 15% achieved HI-E. Among the 74 total patients enrolled, 36 (49%) had prior HMA and 35 (47%) had prior lenalidomide exposure. Twenty-one of 36 patients (58%) who had received previous treatment with HMA achieved HI-E versus 15 of 38 patients (39%) without prior HMA treatment ($P = .10$). Nineteen of 35 patients (54%) who had received previous lenalidomide treatment achieved HI-E versus 17 of 39 patients (44%) without previous lenalidomide treatment ($P = .41$).

On approval, it is hoped that patients with lower-risk MDS with RS will be offered treatment with luspatercept, in particular those with no prior HMA or lenalidomide exposure. Luspatercept will most likely become the standard of care after ESA failure or for patients with low chance of ESA response. Because patients with MDS-RS subtypes have better overall survival, luspatercept will be used for anemic patients who had prior exposure to HMA or lenalidomide, which remains an unmet need.

The underlying biological rationale for better responses in patients with MDS with RS remains unclear. The benefit of treatment may extend well beyond patients with RS. In the PACE study the response rate in the RS-negative patients was 43% (3 out of 7 patients) HI-E and 29% (2 out of 7 patients) became RBC-TI.[21] The HI-E rates in SF3B1 mutated patients were 24 out of 31(77%) and 6 out of 15 (40%) in SF3B1 wild-type patients. The HI-E rate in patients with other splicing mutations was 73% (27 out of 37) compared with 36% (5 out of 14) in patients without splicing mutations.[15] Further studies are needed to explore whether there is a unique mechanism of action for luspatercept in patients with RS or splicing mutations. As a terminal erythroid differentiating agent, the authors hope the benefit and response will fill unmet needs for anemia treatment in LR-MDS for all patients. In practice, luspatercept may become an option for patients after ESA failure and/or lenalidomide/HMA failure. However, further studies in these patients are warranted.

In the MEDALIST study, secondary end point analysis responses were higher among patients with LTB. The Hgb increase of greater than or equal to 1.5 g/dL was reported in 69.6% of patients with less than 4 U/8 wk RBC-TD at baseline treated with luspatercept, and 60% of patients with less than 6 U/8 wk baseline RBC-TD became RBC-TI. The responses were higher among patients within 5 years of MDS diagnosis.[22] This finding may suggest that earlier treatment could be more beneficial. In contrast, the benefit of treatment in HTB patients extends beyond RBC-TI patients, in whom 54% of patients with baseline greater than 4 U/8 wk showed sustained RBC transfusion reduction of 4 U or more.

In the author's practice, if the drug is approved, we will use luspatercept for patients with LR-MDS with RS after ESA failure/intolerance or among those with low chance of response to ESA. We will consider earlier introduction before heavy RBC transfusion dependency. Luspatercept would be an option for those existing patients with MDS-RS after lenalidomide plus HMA failure and a consideration among other patients with non–deletion 5q LR-MDS and no RS.

FUTURE DIRECTIONS

There are many questions to be answered regarding use of luspatercept in MDS. Further exploring whether there is a unique mechanism of action among patients with RS, SF3B1 mutations, or splicing mutations is key. Introducing the treatment earlier among patients with symptomatic anemia or Hgb level less than 9 g/dL before requiring RBC transfusions may be an even more effective strategy. The COMMANDS study is an ongoing randomized clinical trial comparing luspatercept with ESA among all patients with LR-MDS who require at least 2 U RBC transfusion every 8 weeks as an upfront strategy. Combination with ESA, lenalidomide, and HMA in patients with LR-MDS is worth exploring. Use of luspatercept in patients with deletion 5q MDS after lenalidomide failure can be further explored and eventually used as supportive therapy added to HMA-based combinations in higher-risk MDS.

DISCLOSURE

Speaker bureaus: Jazz Pharmaceuticals, Novartis Oncology, Alexion Pharmaceuticals. Consultancy and Advisory boards: Celgene, Novartis Oncology, Jazz Pharmaceuticals, Daiichi-Sankyo, Inc (DSI), Agios Pharmaceuticals, Janssen and Janssen, Pfizer.

REFERENCES

1. Komrokji RS, Sekeres MA, List AF. Management of lower-risk myelodysplastic syndromes: the art and evidence. Curr Hematol Malig Rep 2011;6(2):145–53.
2. Komrokji R, Bennett JM. The myelodysplastic syndromes: classification and prognosis. Curr Hematol Rep 2003;2(3):179–85.
3. Abel GA, Efficace F, Buckstein RJ, et al. Prospective international validation of the Quality of Life in Myelodysplasia Scale (QUALMS). Haematologica 2016;101(6): 781–8.
4. Goldberg SL, Chen E, Sasane M, et al. Economic impact on US Medicare of a new diagnosis of myelodysplastic syndromes and the incremental costs associated with blood transfusion need. Transfusion 2012;52(10):2131–8.
5. Hellstrom-Lindberg E, Gulbrandsen N, Lindberg G, et al. A validated decision model for treating the anaemia of myelodysplastic syndromes with erythropoietin + granulocyte colony-stimulating factor: significant effects on quality of life. Br J Haematol 2003;120(6):1037–46.
6. List A, Dewald G, Bennett J, et al. Lenalidomide in the myelodysplastic syndrome with chromosome 5q deletion. N Engl J Med 2006;355(14):1456–65.
7. Santini V, Almeida A, Giagounidis A, et al. Randomized Phase III Study of Lenalidomide Versus Placebo in RBC Transfusion-Dependent Patients With Lower-Risk Non-del(5q) Myelodysplastic Syndromes and Ineligible for or Refractory to Erythropoiesis-Stimulating Agents. Journal of Clinical Oncology 2016;34(25): 2988–96.
8. Lyons RM, Cosgriff TM, Modi SS, et al. Hematologic response to three alternative dosing schedules of azacitidine in patients with myelodysplastic syndromes. J Clin Oncol 2009;27(11):1850–6.
9. Stahl M, DeVeaux M, de Witte T, et al. The use of immunosuppressive therapy in MDS: clinical outcomes and their predictors in a large international patient cohort. Blood Adv 2018;2(14):1765–72.
10. Blank U, Karlsson S. The role of Smad signaling in hematopoiesis and translational hematology. Leukemia 2011;25:1379.
11. Komrokji RS. Activin receptor II ligand traps: new treatment paradigm for low-risk MDS. Curr Hematol Malig Rep 2019;14(4):346–51.
12. Valent P, Büsche G, Theurl I, et al. Normal and pathological erythropoiesis in adults: from gene regulation to targeted treatment concepts. Haematologica 2018;103(10):1593–603.
13. Zhao B, Liu H, Mei Y, et al. Disruption of erythroid nuclear opening and histone release in myelodysplastic syndromes. Cancer Med 2019;8(3):1169–74.

14. Basiorka AA, McGraw KL, Eksioglu EA, et al. The NLRP3 inflammasome functions as a driver of the myelodysplastic syndrome phenotype. Blood 2016;128(25): 2960–75.

15. Schmierer B, Hill CS. TGF[beta]-SMAD signal transduction: molecular specificity and functional flexibility. Nat Rev Mol Cell Biol 2007;8(12):970–82.

16. Zhou L, Nguyen AN, Sohal D, et al. Inhibition of the TGF-beta receptor I kinase promotes hematopoiesis in MDS. Blood 2008;112(8):3434–43.

17. Zhou L, McMahon C, Bhagat T, et al. Reduced SMAD7 leads to overactivation of TGF-beta signaling in MDS that can be reversed by a specific inhibitor of TGF-beta receptor I kinase. Cancer Res 2011;71(3):955–63.

18. Bhagat TD, Zhou L, Sokol L, et al. miR-21 mediates hematopoietic suppression in MDS by activating TGF-beta signaling. Blood 2013;121(15):2875–81.

19. Suragani RNVS, Cadena SM, Cawley SM, et al. Transforming growth factor-[beta] superfamily ligand trap ACE-536 corrects anemia by promoting late-stage erythropoiesis. Nat Med 2014;20(4):408–14.

20. Attie KM, Allison MJ, McClure T, et al. A phase 1 study of ACE-536, a regulator of erythroid differentiation, in healthy volunteers. Am J Hematol 2014;89(7):766–70.

21. Platzbecker U, Germing U, Götze KS, et al. Luspatercept for the treatment of anaemia in patients with lower-risk myelodysplastic syndromes (PACE-MDS): a multicentre, open-label phase 2 dose-finding study with long-term extension study. Lancet Oncol 2017;18(10):1338–47.

22. Fennaux P, Platzbecker U, Mufti G, et al. The medalist trial: results of a phase 3, randomized, double-blind, placebo-controlled study of luspatercept to treat anemia in patients with very low-, low-, or intermediate-risk Myelodysplastic Syndromes (MDS) with Ring Sideroblasts (RS) Who Require Red Blood Cell (RBC) transfusions. Blood 2018;132(Suppl 1):1.

23. Komrokji R, Garcia-Manero G, Ades L, et al. Sotatercept with long-term extension for the treatment of anaemia in patients with lower-risk myelodysplastic syndromes: a phase 2, dose-ranging trial. Lancet Haematol 2018;5(2):e63–72.

Treatment of Acquired Sideroblastic Anemias

Abhishek A. Mangaonkar, MBBS, Mrinal M. Patnaik, MD*

KEYWORDS

- Ring sideroblast • RS • *SF3B1* • MDS-RS • MDS

KEY POINTS

- Acquired sideroblastic anemias can be categorized into 2 groups: clonal and non-clonal.
- Clonal acquired sideroblastic anemias refer to myeloid neoplasms with ring sideroblasts and are often characterized by somatic alterations in the *SF3B1* gene, which encodes a key protein of the spliceosome U2snRNP complex.
- Anemia is a major cause of morbidity among patients with clonal sideroblastic anemias and therapeutic strategies include erythropoiesis stimulating agents (erythropoietin a or β, darbopoietin α), immunomodulatory agents (lenalidomide), and TGF-β ligand modulators (luspatercept).
- Besides anemia, clonal evolution and thrombosis (increased risk in certain subtypes such as myelodysplastic/myeloproliferative neoplasms with ring sideroblasts and thrombocytosis) are other disease-related complications, while iron overload can be a long-term complication because of ineffective erythropoiesis and red blood cell transfusion dependency.
- Future areas of research include novel strategies for restoration of erythropoiesis such as telomerase inhibition and splicing modulation.

INTRODUCTION

Sideroblastic anemias are characterized by the presence of abnormal erythroid precursors known as ring sideroblasts (RS) in the bone marrow aspirate smear stained by Prussian blue stain (also known as Perls Prussian blue staining technique). Definition of an RS, as per an accepted consensus proposal by the International Working Group (IWG) on Morphology of Myelodysplastic Syndromes (MDS), requires at least 5 siderotic granules covering at least one-third of the nuclear circumference (**Fig. 1**).[1] RS are always found in pathologic states, and are distinct from ferritin sideroblasts, which can be seen in normal bone marrow aspirate evaluations. Unutilized excess iron appears as a few scattered cytoplasmic granules (also known as

Division of Hematology, Department of Medicine, Mayo Clinic, 200 1st Street Southwest, Rochester, MN 55905, USA
* Corresponding author.
E-mail address: Patnaik.Mrinal@mayo.edu

Hematol Oncol Clin N Am 34 (2020) 401–420
https://doi.org/10.1016/j.hoc.2019.11.002
0889-8588/20/© 2019 Elsevier Inc. All rights reserved.

hemonc.theclinics.com

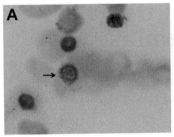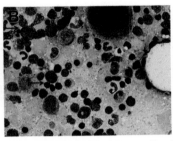

Fig. 1. Panel showing RS and erythroid hyperplasia in MDS-RS. (*A*) Prussian blue stain demonstrating bone marrow ring sideroblasts (*arrow*). (*B*) Wright Giemsa stain demonstrating erythroid hyperplasia (*arrow*). MDS, myelodysplastic; RS, ring sideroblast. (*Courtesy of* J.L. Oliveira, MD, Rochester, MN.)

siderosomes); however, in pathologic states with RS, iron is abnormally stored in the mitochondria. This process is normally regulated by the ferroxidase enzyme encoded by *FTMT* (for expansion of gene names, go to www.genenames.org), an intronless gene on chromosome 5q23.1.[2,3]

Patients with sideroblastic anemias can have a broad range of differential diagnoses, and can be grouped into 2 subtypes, inherited and acquired. Acquired sideroblastic anemias can further be classified into clonal (neoplastic) and nonclonal (nonneoplastic) (**Fig. 2**). This article focuses on the management options for acquired sideroblastic anemias.

ACQUIRED SIDEROBLASTIC ANEMIAS

Acquired sideroblastic anemias can be grouped into clonal and nonclonal subtypes. Clonal sideroblastic anemias are myeloid neoplasms with RS and are often associated with somatic perturbations in the *SF3B1* gene, which encodes a crucial protein of the spliceosome U2snRNP complex. However, patients may also harbor other variants regulating the RNA splicing machinery (such as *U2AF1*, *ZRSR2*, and *SRSF2*), either in isolation, or concomitantly with known myeloid neoplasm-associated variants such as *TET2* and *ASXL1*.[4]

Myeloid neoplasms with RS can be divided into 4 broad categories: myelodysplastic syndromes (MDS), myeloproliferative neoplasms (MPNs), myelodysplastic/myeloproliferative (MDS/MPN) overlap syndromes, and acute myeloid leukemia (AML, see **Fig. 2**). In the 2016 iteration of the World Health Organization (WHO) classification of myeloid neoplasms, there were several changes made to the categories of MDS.[5] Specifically, MDS patients with at least 15% RS (or ≥ 5% RS in the presence of *SF3B1* pathogenic variants [^{mt}]), less than 5% myeloblasts (per nucleated cells) in the bone marrow (BM), and less than 1% of peripheral blood leukocytes, absence of Auer rods, and without fulfilling diagnostic criteria for MDS with isolated del(5q) were grouped into a unified entity called MDS-RS.[5,6] Based on the affected lineages, MDS-RS was further subclassified into single-lineage dysplasia (MDS-RS-SLD) or multilineage dysplasia (MDS-RS-MLD).[5] In the previous WHO classification, MDS-RS-SLD patients were included as refractory anemia with ring sideroblasts (RARS), while MDS-RS-MLD patients were included under RCMD, a category that also included patients with MDS-MLD.[6] However, MDS-RS is not the only category under myeloid neoplasms to include patients with RS and *SF3B1*^{mt}. Myeloid neoplasms such as essential thrombocythemia (ET), primary myelofibrosis (PMF), and MDS/MPN overlap syndromes such as chronic myelomonocytic leukemia (CMML), MDS/

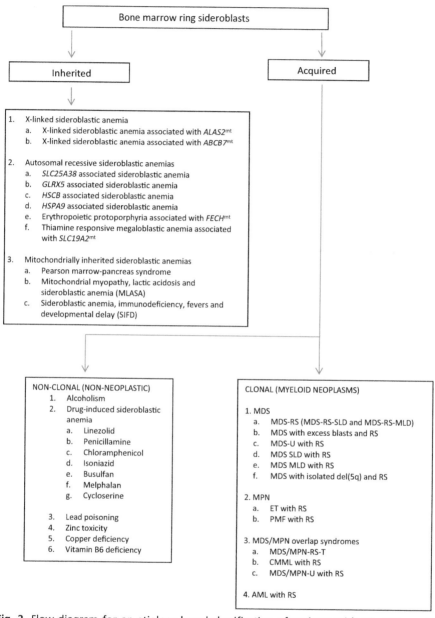

Fig. 2. Flow diagram for an etiology-based classification of patients with RS. AML, acute myeloid leukemia; CMML, chronic myelomonocytic leukemia; ET, essential thrombocythemia; MDS, myelodysplastic syndromes; MLD, multilineage dysplasia; MPN, myeloproliferative neoplasm; PMF, primary myelofibrosis; RS, ring sideroblast; SLD, single lineage dysplasia; T, thrombocytosis; U, unclassifiable.

MPN overlap syndrome with RS and thrombocytosis (MDS/MPN-RS-T), and MDS/MPN, unclassifiable (MDS/MPN-U) can all present with RS with or without $SF3B1^{mt}$.[3,7] Interestingly, BM RS have also been identified in patients with acute myeloid leukemia (AML), where they tend to associate with adverse genetic features such as $TP53^{mt}$.[8]

In MDS patients without excess blasts, BM RS percentage has not been found to be prognostically relevant, both for overall (OS) and leukemia-free survival (LFS), resulting in the recent 2016 WHO criteria modification, allowing inclusion of MDS patients with at least 5% RS and $SF3B1^{mt}$ as 'MDS-RS'.[9] Literature with regards to the prognostic relevance of $SF3B1^{mt}$ in MDS is controversial, with some studies,[7,10] but not all,[11–13] reporting an independent favorable prognostic impact. However, in the context of classifying MDS-RS into morphologic subtypes based on affected lineages (MDS-RS-SLD and MDS-RS-MLD), molecular information such as absence of $SF3B1^{mt}$ and presence of $ASXL1^{mt}$ were found to independently predict adverse outcomes.[14] In other words, although there were no differences in outcomes (both OS and LFS) among patients with MDS-RS-SLD and MDS-RS-MLD, the presence of $SF3B1^{mt}$ and absence of $ASXL1^{mt}$ were found to independently predict favorable outcomes and remained relevant in the context of the revised International Prognostic Scoring System (R-IPSS) risk stratification.[14,15] This data calls into question the relevance of morphology-based classification of MDS-RS and makes a strong case for incorporating molecular aberrations in future revisions of the WHO classification.

NONCLONAL ACQUIRED SIDEROBLASTIC ANEMIAS

Nonclonal, acquired sideroblastic anemias usually arise as a consequence of nutritional defects or ingestion/accumulation of toxins and can be seen in the context of alcohol abuse and associated pyridoxine deficiency.[16] Alternative causes include copper deficiency[17] and drugs such as isoniazid (secondary to pyridoxine deficiency), chloramphenicol, linezolid, penicillamine, busulfan, melphalan, and cycloserine (see **Fig. 2**).[3,18,19] Heme synthesis in the mitochondria depends on pyridoxal phosphate (activated pyridoxine), which functions as a cofactor for enzyme 5-aminolevulinate (ALA) synthase and produces a precursor of heme (ALA) in a single, rate-limiting step.[20] Disruption of this process results in locking of iron in the mitochondria, thereby causing anemia and bone marrow RS, thus explaining the responses sometimes seen with pyridoxine replacement.[20]

MANAGEMENT

Management of acquired sideroblastic anemias depends on the etiology. Clonally derived myeloid neoplasms with RS merit a risk-adapted individualized approach. Patients at a higher risk of transformation into AML need to be considered for potentially curative strategies such as allogeneic hematopoietic stem cell transplantation (HSCT), while patients with lower-risk disease need appropriate supportive care strategies to lower morbidity and long-term complications such as iron overload.

Clonal Sideroblastic Anemias

Anemia

In myeloid neoplasms associated with RS, anemia is thought to be secondary to ineffective erythropoiesis and an accelerated rate of progenitor cell Fas-triggered apoptosis in the bone marrow.[21,22] Because of increasing transfusion need and complications from secondary hemochromatosis (iron overload), anemia is a significant cause of increased morbidity and reduced quality of life.[23,24] Several therapies have been successful in treating anemic patients with myeloid neoplasms and RS

Erythropoiesis stimulation: Erythropoiesis stimulating agents (ESAs) have successfully been used to decrease the red blood cell (RBC) transfusion need and to improve quality of life in patients with MDS-RS and suboptimal endogenous erythropoietin responses (EPO <500 Mu/L).[23,25] Response rates among ESA-naïve MDS patients are estimated to range from 45% to 73%, with lower responses (25%–75%) in those previously treated with ESAs. Most responses occur within 8 weeks of treatment, with a median duration of approximately 24 months.[3,26] Although data are conflicting, at least a few studies confirm higher responses to ESA therapy for patients with MDS-RS-SLD compared with other MDS subtypes.[27,28] Biologically, whether ESA responses occur through proliferation of dysplastic clone or normal erythropoiesis remains a matter of debate. Clinically, there is no convincing evidence of increased progression to AML upon ESA use or upon addition of G-CSF.[26]

Response to ESA depends on several factors such as pretreatment transfusion need and baseline serum EPO level.[25,29] Major predictors of response include EPO level of no more than 500 U/L and less than 2 units/month of RBC transfusion need, while presence of only one of these factors predicts for an intermediate response.[25] Alternative predictors include bone marrow blast less than 10%, normal cytogenetics, lower (low or intermediate) risk IPSS subtype, and shorter duration of disease.[30] In clinical practice, a trial of ESA is usually not recommended among patients with an endogenous EPO level greater than 500 U/L.

There are several published randomized and single arm clinical trials, and prospective studies assessing the efficacy of ESA in MDS reviewed in detail elsewhere.[26] Among the randomized clinical trials (**Table 1**), erythroid responses (HI-E) as assessed by the 2006 IWG criteria (defined as persistent [$\geq$8 weeks] improvement of pretreatment hemoglobin < 11 g/dL by at least $\geq$ 1.5 gm/dL, or relevant reduction of RBC transfusion units by an absolute number of at least 4 every 8 weeks)[31] to ESA range in between 30% and 35%.[3] The first published randomized study assessing erythropoietin α (EA) randomized 110 patients with MDS (RARS, n = 30) to EA (150 U/kg daily) plus supportive care (SC) versus SC alone, and erythroid responses at 4 months (as assessed by the 2006 IWG response criteria) were found to be significantly higher in the EA group (34 vs 5.8%, P=.001), with subgroup analysis showing higher responses in the RA and RARS group versus the RAEB group (45 vs 10%, P=.006).[27] Two other placebo-controlled phase 3 studies assessing efficacy of EA versus placebo confirmed higher erythroid responses with EA; however, responses were not significantly different among patients with RS.[32,33] Fenaux and colleagues[32] reported a phase 3, placebo-controlled study where 130 patients with IPSS low- or intermediate-1 risk MDS (RARS 4.4%, RCMD-RS 11.1%) were randomized in a 2:1 manner to receive EA at a dose of 450 IU/kg/wk (n = 85) versus placebo (n = 45). At 24 weeks, patients in the EA arm had higher erythroid responses as assessed by the 2006 IWG response criteria (31.8 vs 4.4%, P<.001), while responses did not differ in the RARS/RCMD-RS subtypes.[32] Another phase 3 placebo-control trial randomized 131 MDS (RARS 15.3%) patients to EA at 150 U/kg/d versus placebo. At 8 weeks, responses in the EA group were higher (36.8 vs 10.8%, P=.007).[33] Darbopoietin α (DA) is an alternative erythropoietin formulation with approximately three-fold longer half-life as opposed to recombinant human erythropoietins such as EA.[34] A phase 3 trial randomized (2:1 method) 147 IPSS low-/intermediate-1 risk MDS patients to DA versus placebo and found higher responses in the DA group versus placebo (14.7 vs 0%, P=.016) at 24 weeks as per the IWG 2006 criteria, with no significant differences among patients with RARS.[35] Most responses to ESA occur within 8 weeks of therapy and require careful observation to ensure that the hemoglobin levels do not increase beyond 11 gm/dL, as this can be associated with complications such as venous thromboembolism, hypertension, and worsening systolic heart failure.[3]

DA and EA have not been directly compared in a randomized clinical trial, although meta-analyses have not demonstrated any significant clinical differences between the

Table 1
Randomized phase 3 clinical trials assessing erythropoiesis-stimulating agent use in low-risk myelodysplastic syndromes

ESA Type	Type of Study	ESA Dose	Number of Patients	Erythroid Response	References
Darbopoietin alpha (DA)	Phase 3, placebo control arm	500 μg every 3 weeks (frequency could be increased to 2 weeks in the 48-wk open-label phase)	147 (RARS 14.4%) randomized 2:1 to DA (n = 98) or placebo (n = 49)	At 24 weeks, HI-E (IWG 2006 criteria[a]) achieved: DA vs placebo (14.7 vs 0%, P=.016); 22% (2/9) in RARS. At 48 weeks, end of blinded treatment and all patients received DA, overall HI-E 34.7% (RARS-35%) (28.9% prior placebo vs 26.4% prior DA)	Platzbecker et al,[35] 2017
Epoetin-alpha (EA)	Phase 3, placebo control arm	450 IU/kg/wk	130 (RARS 4.4%, RCMD-RS 11.1%) Randomized 2:1 to EA (n = 85) or placebo (n = 45)	At 24 weeks, erythroid response as per IWG 2006 criteria: EA vs placebo (31.8 vs 4.4%, P<.001); 38.1% in RARS/RCMD-RS	Fenaux et al,[32] 2018

Epoetin-alpha (EA)	Phase 3, placebo control arm	131 (RARS 15.3%) randomized 1:1 to EA and placebo	150 U/kg/d in the 8-wk double-blind phase (as per response, both drug and placebo groups received EA at 150–300 U/kg three times per week in the open week starting at 24 weeks)	As predefined response criteria[b] Full plus partial responses: EA vs placebo (36.8 vs 10.8%, $P=.007$); in RARS: 37.5 vs 18.2% ($P=.6$)	Ferrini et al,[33] 1998
Epoetin-alpha (EA)	Phase 3, supportive care (SC) control arm	110 (RARS, n = 30) randomized to EPO + SC (n = 53) vs SC (n = 57)	150 U/kg daily	At 4 mo evaluation, IWG 2006 response criteria, EA plus SC versus SC only (34 vs 5.8%, $P=.001$); in RA and RARS, response rate was higher than RAEB (45 vs 10%, $P=.006$)	Greenberg et al,[27] 2009

Abbreviations: ESA, erythropoiesis stimulating agent; HI-E, erythroid response; IWG, international working group; MDS, myelodysplastic syndromes; RAEB, refractory anemia with excess blasts; RARS, refractory anemia with ring sideroblasts; RCMD, refractory cytopenia with multilineage dysplasia; RS, ring sideroblast.

[a] IWG 2006 erythroid response: Persistent ($\geq$8 weeks) improvement of pretreatment hemoglobin less than 11 g/dL by at least $\geq$ 1.5 gm/dL or relevant reduction of units of RBC transfusions by an absolute number of at least 4 RBC transfusions every 8 weeks compared with the pretreatment transfusion number in the previous 8 weeks. Only transfusions.

[b] Full response defined as increased in hemoglobin $\geq$ 2 gm/dL (2 consecutive controls in the same week) or no transfusion for at least 2 months; partial response defined as increase in Hb of 1 to 2 gm/dL (2 consecutive controls in the same week) or 50% decrease in transfusion need for at least 2 months; no response defined as Hb change less than 1 gm/dL or less than 50% reduction of transfusion requirements.

2 drugs.[30,36,37] Combining ESA with G-CSF may have long-lasting higher erythroid responses without any significant risk of accelerated progression to AML as shown by the long-term follow-up of patients from the Nordic MDS group studies.[38]

Immunomodulatory agents: Lenalidomide is an immunomodulatory agent with preferential activity among MDS patients with isolated del (5q) by inducing degradation of casein kinase 1A1 (CK1α) in a cereblon (CRBN)-dependent manner, which preferentially affects del (5q) cells because of CK1α haploinsufficiency.[39] In a pivotal phase 3, randomized, placebo-controlled clinical trial, lenalidomide was shown to decrease RBC transfusion requirement (RBC transfusion independence [TI] ≥ 8 weeks) in patients with IPSS lower-risk non del (5q) MDS (26.9 vs 2.5%, $P<.001$).[40] There was significant preferential response among MDS patients with RS, although only 7.5% of patients carried a diagnosis of RARS.[40] Median time to onset of response was 10.1 weeks, with 90% patients achieving RBC-TI for at least 8 weeks. In a multivariate analysis, low RBC transfusion burden (< 4 units/28 days) and prior use of ESA before study inclusion were found to be independent prognostic indicators for achieving erythroid response. Interestingly, although serum EPO level of no more than 500 mU/mL was a significant prognostic factor for achieving RBC-TI in greater than or equal to 8 weeks in a univariate analysis, it did not hold significance in a multivariate model. Significant treatment-emergent adverse effects included neutropenia, thrombocytopenia, diarrhea, infection, and bleeding. Three percent of patients developed venous thromboembolism, while 2.5% patients developed arterial thromboembolism.[40] A phase 2 study for RBC transfusion-dependent (TD) lower-risk MDS patients with karyotypes other than del(5q) reported 35% erythroid responses to lenalidomide among RARS patients.[41]

Addition of lenalidomide to ESA may show a synergistic effect, even in patients who are otherwise refractory or ineligible for ESA therapy. A European phase III study randomized 131 RBC transfusion-dependent, ESA-refractory, lower-risk MDS (RARS 39.7%, RCMD-RS 25.4%) non-del(5q) patients to receive lenalidomide alone at 10 mg per day for 21 days every 4 weeks, or lenalidomide at the same dosing schedule with EPO β at 60,000 U per week. In an intention-to-treat (ITT) analysis, higher rates of erythroid response (39.4 vs 23.1%, $P=.044$) were seen in the combination arm versus lenalidomide alone.[42] Correlative studies demonstrated low baseline EPO levels and G polymorphism in the *CRBN* gene as predictors of response.[42] These findings were confirmed in the United States through the Eastern Cooperative Group E2905 trial, which randomized ESA-refractory low- or intermediate-1 IPSS risk MDS patients to either lenalidomide (10 mg/d for 21 days every 4 weeks) plus EA (60,000 U per week) versus lenalidomide alone and found a higher rate of 2006 IWG-defined major erythroid response in the former group (25.6 vs 9.9%, $P=.015$).[43] These studies highlight the possibility of overcoming ESA resistance by the addition of lenalidomide in a sizable proportion of patients.

Retrospective case series have demonstrated erythroid responses to lenalidomide in both transfusion-dependent MDS-RS and MDS/MPN-RS-T.[44,45] In a clinically and molecularly annotated Mayo Clinic cohort of 357 MDS patients, patients with *SF3B1*[mt] were more likely to respond to lenalidomide than *SF3B1* wild-type patients (56 vs 27%, $P=.04$).[46] Among non-TD MDS patients, lenalidomide use did not improve OS, suggesting that the drug's benefit is limited to improving anemia without any overall effect on disease modification.[47]

TGF-β ligand modulation: The TGF-β superfamily consists of several growth factors and proteins, including activatory and inhibitory SMAD proteins, capable of negatively regulating hematopoietic stem cell proliferation and differentiation.[21] Abnormalities in TGF- β have been implicated as a cause of suppressed erythropoiesis in lower-risk

MDS and inhibitors such as luspatercept (ACE-536, a novel recombinant fusion protein containing modified activin receptor type IIb tied to the Fc domain of human immunoglobulin G1)[48] and sotatercept (ACE-011, a recombinant human fusion protein containing the extracellular domain of activin receptor IIA)[49] have been successfully developed to modulate this pathway. A study of luspatercept to treat anemia caused by very low-, low-, or intermediate- risk MDS (MEDALIST) trial was a phase 3, randomized, double-blind, placebo-controlled study that randomized 229 patients with lower-risk, TD, ESA-refractory or intolerant, MDS-RS in a 2:1 manner to receive either luspatercept at 1 mg/kg administered subcutaneously every 21 days (n = 153), or placebo (n = 76), with the primary end point being RBC TI for at least 8 weeks. Higher rates of response were observed in the luspatercept group compared with placebo (37.9 vs 13.2%, $P<.0001$), with minimal toxicities or evidence for disease progression.[50] In a prior phase 2, open-label PACE-MDS study that included 58 IPSS-defined low- or intermediate-1 risk MDS patients, IWG erythroid response was achieved by 63% patients receiving luspatercept, while RBC-TI was achieved by 38% patients.[48] Grade 3 adverse effects included myalgia (2%), while grade 1 to 2 adverse effects were fatigue (7%), bone pain (5%), diarrhea (5%), and headaches (3%).[48] Sotatercept has been studied in a phase 2, open-label trial that randomized 74 patients with R-IPSS-defined low- or intermediate-risk, TD, ESA-refractory, or intolerant MDS-RS. Forty nine percent of patients achieved the primary end point of HI-E as defined by the 2006 IWG MDS response assessment criteria (**Table 2**).[51] An ongoing study is assessing luspatercept versus ESA in the frontline setting, in TD, ESA-naïve lower-risk MDS patients (NCT03682536).

Telomerase inhibition: Imetelstat is a lipid-conjugated oligonucleotide that targets the RNA template of human telomerase reverse transcriptase. In a pilot phase 2 study, imetelstat was shown to have single-agent activity in myelofibrosis.[52] Among myelofibrosis patients with $SF3B1^{mt}$ or $U2AF1^{mt}$, complete clinical and molecular remissions were observed. This led to another study that included 9 MDS patients with RS, RARS-T (n = 5), RARS (n = 3), and myelodysplastic/myeloproliferative neoplasm with a spliceosome mutation (n = 1).[53] Three (38%) of 8 TD patients became transfusion independent after a median time of 11 weeks, lasting for a median of 28 weeks, suggesting single-agent activity in myeloid neoplasm patients with RS.[53] Results from a larger phase 2/3 trial that studied imetelstat at a dose of 7.5 mg/kg every 4 weeks in 38 patients with TD, low- or intermediate-1 IPSS risk, ESA-refractory, or intolerant MDS patients indicated a robust erythroid response, with 37% achieving RBC-TI for at least 8 weeks (33% in RARS/RCMD-RS patients).[54] Significant toxicities include neutropenia and thrombocytopenia (grade ≥ 3 in 58% patients), and hepatic transaminitis (mostly grade 1 or 2) (see **Table 2**). Although results appear promising, results from randomized phase 3 trials are awaited.

Splicing inhibition: Heterozygous mutations in genes affecting splicing (SF3B1, U2AF1, and SRSF2) are common in myeloid neoplasms with RS. These mutations cause the clonal cells to rely on their wild-type allele for splicing function, which can be therapeutically targeted to achieve synthetic lethality.[55] H3B-8800 is an orally available small molecular splicing modulator that utilizes the aforementioned mechanism to preferentially kill spliceosome mutant cells.[55] Results from prospective clinical trials are awaited (NCT02841540).

Other agents: Anabolic steroids such as danazol or oxymetholone have been shown to improve anemia in retrospective cohorts of MDS patients; however, adverse effects such as hepatic transminitis, dyslipidemia, and prostate hyperplasia need close

Table 2
Novel drugs in the treatment of clonal sideroblastic anemias

Drug and Dose	Mechanism of Action	Type of Study	Number of Patients	Response	References
Luspatercept, 1 mg/kg subcutaneously every 21 d	First-in-class erythroid maturation agent, TGF-β pathway modulation	Phase 3, randomized, placebo controlled	229 patients with R-IPSS low- or intermediate-risk, TD, ESA refractory or intolerant MDS-RS randomized 2:1 to receive luspatercept (n = 153) or placebo (n = 76)	RBC-TI ≥ 8 weeks (primary end point): luspatercept vs placebo (37.9 vs 13.2%, P<.0001)	Fenaux et al,[50] 2018
Sotatercept, 0.1 or 0.3 mg/kg every 21 d	Activin receptor type IIA fusion protein, TGF-β pathway modulation	Phase 2, open-label	74 patients with R-IPSS low or intermediate-risk, TD, ESA refractory or intolerant MDS-RS	HI-E as per IWG 2006 criteria (primary endpoint): 36/74 (49%) achieved the primary end point	Komrokji et al,[51] 2018
Imetelstat, 7.5 mg/kg intravenously every 4 weeks	Telomerase inhibition	Phase 2/3	38 TD, Low-risk MDS, refractory or intolerant to ESA, lenalidomide/ HMA naïve	RBC-TI ≥ 8 wk (primary endpoint): (14/38) 37%; RARS/RCMD-RS (33%)	Steensma et al,[54] 2018
H3B-8800, optimal dose not yet established	Splicing modulation	Open-label, phase 1 trial ongoing	MDS, AML and CMML	N/A	Seiler et al,[55] 2018

Abbreviations: ESA, erythropoiesis stimulating agent; HI-E, erythroid response; IWG, international working group; MDS, myelodysplastic syndromes; RARS, refractory anemia with ring sideroblasts; RBC-TI, red blood cell transfusion independence; RCMD, refractory cytopenia with multilineage dysplasia; R-IPSS, revised international prognostic scoring system; RS, ring sideroblast; TD, transfusion dependent.

monitoring.[29,56,57] Eltrombopag has also been used in patients with lower-risk MDS, with improvements in platelet counts and in a minority of patients, improvement in hemoglobin levels. However, studies have raised a concern for accelerated clonal evolution and progression to AML and rigorous prospective validation for the use of this agent is still needed.[58,59]

Iron chelation therapy

In general, patients with myeloid neoplasms and RS have an indolent disease course because of favorable molecular and cytogenetic risk profiles.[3,14,15] As iterated before, TD anemia remains a significant cause of morbidity, with secondary hemochromatosis (iron overload) being a major complication. Iron status can be monitored through laboratory tests such as serum ferritin, transferrin saturation, and by utilization of T2* cardiac and liver MRI scans, thereby obviating the need for invasive tests such as a liver biopsy.[3] In addition, early evidence of hepatic fibrosis/cirrhosis can be detected by using Fibroscans (ultrasound-based) and MR Elastograms.[60]

Several iron chelators are currently available for the treatment of transfusion iron overload in myeloid neoplasms with RS, including parenteral (deferoxamine) and oral (deferasirox and deferiprone) agents. However, all of these agents are associated with potential severe adverse effects necessitating a careful risk-benefit assessment prior to initiation.[61] Deferasirox has been associated with elevation of serum creatinine (36%), hepatic transaminitis (2%), and gastrointestinal (GI) adverse effects such as nausea and diarrhea (8.8%).[60] Deferiprone has been associated with GI adverse effects (33%) and agranulocytosis (1%), while deferoxamine, usually used in children with congenital hemolytic anemias, has been associated with deafness (32.8%), growth retardation (70%), and visual side effects (9.9%).[60] The TELESTO trial was a phase 2, double-blind study that randomized 225 adult patients with IPSS low-/intermediate-1 risk MDS with iron overload to receive either deferasirox (10–40 mg/kg/d per dosing guidelines) or placebo.[62] Participants were also required to have a transfusion history of receiving between 15 and 75 PRBC units, have a serum ferritin level greater than 1000 ng/mL, and be free from cardiac, liver, and renal abnormalities.[62] Results showed that although the serum ferritin levels declined with deferasirox therapy, along with a higher event-free survival, there was no demonstrated difference in OS, possibly an artifact of premature study discontinuation and subsequent iron chelation therapy.[62]

The National Comprehensive Cancer Network (NCCN) guidelines recommend consideration of once-daily deferoxamine subcutaneously or deferasirox orally in the patients with IPSS low- or intermediate-1 risk MDS, with either serum ferritin levels greater than 2500 ng/mL, or in those who have received or anticipated to receive more than 20 units PRBC transfusions.[63] The European Leukemia Net (ELN) recommends consideration of iron chelation therapy among TD patients with RA, RARS, or MDS with serum ferritin levels greater than 1000 ng/mL, with PRBC transfusion history of at least 25 units and among patients who are candidates for allogeneic HSCT.[64] Because of potential adverse effects and inconclusive benefits with regards to survival, prospective trial validation and quality-of-life assessment studies are necessary before recommending the routine use of iron chelation therapy in MDS-RS.[3,61]

Hypomethylating agent therapy

In myeloid neoplasms with RS, use of hypomethylating agents (HMAs) such as 5-azacitidine (AZA) or decitabine (DAC) is uncommon in the upfront setting because of a favorable risk profile and lower risk for clonal evolution. However, in patients who are ESA refractory or intolerant, or those who develop signs of disease progression as evidenced by a rising BM blast percentage, or acquisition of additional cytogenetic or molecular abnormalities, HMA therapy can be considered. Pivotal clinical trials that led to the US Food and Drug Administration (FDA) approval of AZA reported erythroid response rates of approximately 40% in MDS patients with RS, but demonstrated no OS advantage or decrease in rates of leukemic transformation. This limits enthusiasm for upfront use of these drugs in these patients.[3,65] However, HMA use can be considered in patients who develop ESA resistance.

A phase 2 study randomized 98 lower-risk, ESA-refractory MDS patients to receive AZA plus EPO-β or AZA alone. In an ITT analysis, RBC-TI after 6 cycles was achieved in 8 (16.3%) patients in the AZA arm and 7 (14.3%) patients in the AZA plus EPO arm ($P=1.0$) without any significant differences in response rates or OS in the 2 arms.[66] Another phase 2 study, randomized R-IPSS defined low- or interedmiate-1 risk MDS patients to receive low-dose DAC in 2 schedules (20 mg/m^2/d for 3 days every 28 days or 20 mg/m^2 on days 1, 8, and 15 every 28 days), with both schedules demonstrating similar efficacy and safety.[67] Another study prospectively assessed low-dose AZA (75 mg/m^2 daily) or low-dose DAC (20 mg/m^2) for 3 consecutive days every 28 days in patients with lower-risk MDS and MDS/MPN overlap syndrome and found higher overall responses in the DAC arm (70 vs 49%, $P=.03$) but no significant difference in RBC-TI rates (32 vs 16%, $P=.2$).[68]

DAC is not orally bioavailable because of the rapid clearance of DAC by an enzyme, cytidine deaminase, in the gut and liver. However, a fixed-dose combination of oral DAC with cedazuridine (novel cytidine deaminase inhibitor) may provide an alternative to parenteral administrations.[69] Second-generation oral HMAs such as guadecitabine (SGI-110) are also being prospectively evaluated in higher-risk MDS and AML, and are expected to be studied in lower-risk MDS patients too.[70]

Immunosuppressive therapy

A large international multicenter cohort of 207 MDS patients (5.1% RARS, 14% SF3B1^{mt}) was examined for predictors of response and outcomes with IST, most commonly antithymocyte globulin (ATG) plus prednisone (steroid monotherapy was excluded). Overall response rate was 48.8%, with 11.2% achieving complete remission (CR), 5.6% partial remission (PR), and 30% RBC-TI.[71] Contrary to previously reported case series, age, TD, paroxysmal nocturnal hemoglobinuria (PNH), or large granular lymphocyte clone and HLA DR15 positivity did not predict response to immunosuppressive therapy (IST).[29] Information about other known response predictors such as BCOR^{mt} or BCORL1^{mt} was not available. Achievement of RBC TI was associated with BM hypoceullarity (cellularity <20%), with horse ATG plus cyclosporine outperforming rabbit ATG or ATG without cyclosporine. In a univariate analysis, patients with SF3B1^{mt} were associated with a suboptimal response rate, but this did not hold true in a multivariate assessment.[71] Prospective trial validation is necessary before routinely recommending IST in lower-risk MDS.[29] In MDS patients with a hypocellular BM at diagnosis, thorough assessment for germline variants-associated delayed-onset inherited bone marrow failure syndromes is necessary before treatment with immunosuppressive drugs.[72–75]

Allogeneic HSCT

Allogeneic HSCT is the only currently available therapy capable of achieving a cure in chronic myeloid neoplasms, but at the cost of substantial treatment-associated morbidity and mortality. As most clonal sideroblastic anemias belong in one of the lower-risk MDS categories, allogeneic HSCT is often not indicated as the first choice of therapy. Cutler and colleagues[76] compared timing of transplant among newly diagnosed MDS patients (age < 60 years) and found that delayed transplantation (at an interval between diagnosis but prior to leukemic progression) was associated with best outcomes for patients with low- and intermediate-1 IPSS groups. Similarly, in another study among older adults (age 60–70 years) with de novo MDS, nontransplantation strategies versus reduced intensity conditioning (RIC) transplantation were associated with favorable OS (77 vs 38 months) and quality-of-life outcomes.[77] Both studies were analyses of large retrospective MDS and transplant cohorts, and results should therefore be interpreted with caution. Consensus expert panel guidelines recommend upfront HSCT consideration for IPSS-defined lower-risk MDS patients with a good performance status and with specific poor risk features such as adverse cytogenetics, persistent blast increase (either by >50% or >15% BM blasts), life-threatening cytopenias, higher PRBC transfusion need (>2 units per month for 6 months), or adverse molecular features.[78] In the absence of the aforementioned poor risk features, nontransplant interventions should be considered first, and HSCT is only recommended after their failure.[78]

Management of thrombosis

Patients with certain subtypes of clonal sideroblastic anemias such as MDS/MPN-RS-T have a propensity to develop thrombotic events at a rate similar to ET (3.6 vs 4.9/100 patients/year) but higher than MDS-RS (3.6 vs 0.9/100 patients/year).[79] This indicates that the thrombotic risk may be related to thrombocytosis and not a direct pathologic consequence of alterations in *SF3B1* gene or RS. However, in a small series of patients with RARS-T (n = 15), thrombotic events occurred only among patients with *SF3B1*[mt] (60%) versus *SF3B1* wildtype patients.[80] This association between *SF3B1*[mt] and thrombosis in MDS/MPN-RS-T needs further investigation. The rate of thrombosis in MDS/MPN-RS-T at any time in the disease course is estimated to be approximately 20%; however, thrombotic events occurring either at or before diagnosis, or after diagnosis, did not impact overall survival in a Mayo Clinic study.[81] As of yet, there are no data on primary thrombosis prophylaxis among patients with MDS/MPN-RS-T. However, among patients with other risk factors for thrombosis such as advanced age (≥60 years), smoking, and cardiovascular risk factors, antiplatelet and cytoreductive strategies similar to ET could be considered.[82]

Nonclonal Acquired Sideroblastic Anemias

Treatment for nonclonal acquired sideroblastic anemias depends on the etiology. Most causes are related to exogenous exposure to offending agents such as alcohol, drugs (eg, linezolid, penicillamine, chloramphenicol, isoniazid, busulfan, melphalan, or cycloserine), lead, or zinc; therefore, stopping the offending the agent is the first step of management. Vitamin B6 and copper deficiency (could be related to zinc excess) are other causes for which appropriate replacement therapy is warranted. Although specific inherited sideroblastic anemias such as those associated with X-linked *ALAS2* variant are responsive to pyridoxine therapy, it is unclear whether the same is true for patients with nonclonal acquired sideroblastic anemia without pyridoxine deficiency.[83] If stopping the offending agent or correction of the underlying deficiency does not reverse the anemia after a few months (≥3 months), and a clonal process is conclusively ruled out, a trial of pyridoxine is reasonable.

FUTURE DIRECTIONS

Although data from clinical trials for novel drugs such as telomerase and splicing inhibitors are awaited, other genomically defined therapies deserve consideration.

Ivosidenib (IDH1 inhibitor) and enasidenib (IDH-2 inhibitor) are specific IDH inhibitors that can be considered for patients with myeloid neoplasms with RS and concomitant *IDH1^mt* or *IDH2^mt*, which co-occur at a frequency of 2% to 5%.[14,84–86] Because of the relative genetic heterogeneity in myeloid neoplasms, future therapies should look at targeting novel pathways instead of inhibition of single mutant genes. One such example is autophagy, which has been implicated as a mechanism by which *SF3B1^mt*

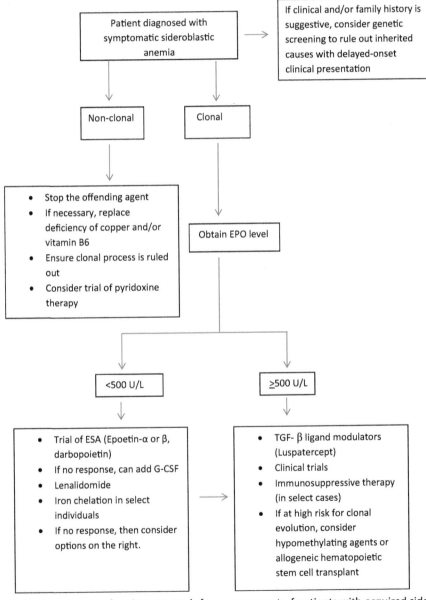

Fig. 3. Flow diagram showing approach for management of patients with acquired sideroblastic anemias. EPO, erythropoietin; ESA, erythropoiesis-stimulating agent; G-CSF, granulocyte colony stimulating factor; TGF-β, transforming growth factor-β.

MDS-RS cells eliminate damaged mitochondria and alleviate toxic effects from iron overload.[87]

SUMMARY OF APPROACH FOR MANAGEMENT OF SIDEROBLASTIC ANEMIAS

Management for sideroblastic anemias depends greatly on appropriate diagnostic and prognostication strategies (**Fig. 3**). It is important to consider genetic screening among patients with a suggestive family history to rule out inherited causes of sideroblastic anemias caused by treatment implications such as pyridoxine responsiveness.[83] Treatments of nonclonal causes depend on the etiology and include either stopping the offending agent (drugs or toxins) or replacement of underlying deficiency (vitamin B6, copper). Treatment of clonal causes is complex and needs a personalized approach for management. Because anemia is the most common cause of morbidity in these patients, restoration of erythropoiesis and achieving RBC TI are the treatment goals in most patients. If ESA therapy is indicated (EPO level <500), a trial of ESA either by itself or in combination of G-CSF or lenalidomide is often successful in improving hemoglobin levels and in reducing RBC transfusion need. The advent of TGF-B modulators such as luspatercept and sotatercept has expanded the inventory of drugs capable of reversing arrested erythropoiesis and can be considered after ESA and/ or lenalidomide failure (currently waiting FDA approval). In later stages of disease, complications such as clonal evolution and iron overload related to repeated RBC transfusions dictate treatment decisions. Although enrollment in clinical trials is preferred, HMAs such as DAC or AZA (including low-dose approaches), IST, and in select individuals, allogeneic HSCT (in select individuals) can be considered (see **Fig. 3**). Novel therapeutic strategies for restoration of effective erythropoiesis, reducing complications from iron overload, and in mitigating clonal evolution are much needed.

ACKNOWLEDGMENTS

The authors would like to acknowledge Dr. Jennifer L. Oliveira, MD, for providing bone marrow biopsy images in **Fig. 1**.

DISCLOSURE

The authors have nothing to disclose.

REFERENCES

1. Mufti GJ, Bennett JM, Goasguen J, et al. Diagnosis and classification of myelodysplastic syndrome: International Working Group on Morphology of myelodysplastic syndrome (IWGM-MDS) consensus proposals for the definition and enumeration of myeloblasts and ring sideroblasts. Haematologica 2008;93(11): 1712–7.
2. Cazzola M, Invernizzi R, Bergamaschi G, et al. Mitochondrial ferritin expression in erythroid cells from patients with sideroblastic anemia. Blood 2003;101(5): 1996–2000.
3. Patnaik MM, Tefferi A. Refractory anemia with ring sideroblasts (RARS) and RARS with thrombocytosis: "2019 update on diagnosis, risk-stratification, and management.". Am J Hematol 2019;94(4):475–88.
4. Patnaik MM, Tefferi A. Refractory anemia with ring sideroblasts (RARS) and RARS with thrombocytosis (RARS-T): 2017 update on diagnosis, risk-stratification, and management. Am J Hematol 2017;92(3):297–310.

5. Arber DA, Orazi A, Hasserjian R, et al. The 2016 revision to the World Health Organization classification of myeloid neoplasms and acute leukemia. Blood 2016; 127(20):2391–405.

6. Vardiman JW, Thiele J, Arber DA, et al. The 2008 revision of the World Health Organization (WHO) classification of myeloid neoplasms and acute leukemia: rationale and important changes. Blood 2009;114(5):937–51.

7. Malcovati L, Karimi M, Papaemmanuil E, et al. SF3B1 mutation identifies a distinct subset of myelodysplastic syndrome with ring sideroblasts. Blood 2015;126(2): 233–41.

8. Martin-Cabrera P, Jeromin S, Perglerova K, et al. Acute myeloid leukemias with ring sideroblasts show a unique molecular signature straddling secondary acute myeloid leukemia and de novo acute myeloid leukemia. Haematologica 2017; 102(4):e125–8.

9. Patnaik MM, Hanson CA, Sulai NH, et al. Prognostic irrelevance of ring sideroblast percentage in World Health Organization-defined myelodysplastic syndromes without excess blasts. Blood 2012;119(24):5674–7.

10. Malcovati L, Papaemmanuil E, Bowen DT, et al. Clinical significance of SF3B1 mutations in myelodysplastic syndromes and myelodysplastic/myeloproliferative neoplasms. Blood 2011;118(24):6239–46.

11. Patnaik MM, Lasho TL, Hodnefield JM, et al. SF3B1 mutations are prevalent in myelodysplastic syndromes with ring sideroblasts but do not hold independent prognostic value. Blood 2012;119(2):569–72.

12. Bejar R, Stevenson K, Abdel-Wahab O, et al. Clinical effect of point mutations in myelodysplastic syndromes. N Engl J Med 2011;364(26):2496–506.

13. Bejar R, Stevenson KE, Caughey BA, et al. Validation of a prognostic model and the impact of mutations in patients with lower-risk myelodysplastic syndromes. J Clin Oncol 2012;30(27):3376–82.

14. Mangaonkar AA, Lasho TL, Finke CM, et al. Prognostic interaction between bone marrow morphology and SF3B1 and ASXL1 mutations in myelodysplastic syndromes with ring sideroblasts. Blood Cancer J 2018;8(2):18.

15. Mangaonkar AA, Gangat N, Al-Kali A, et al. Prognostic impact of ASXL1 mutations in patients with myelodysplastic syndromes and multilineage dysplasia with or without ring sideroblasts. Leuk Res 2018;71:60–2.

16. Tenner S, Rollhauser C, Butt F, et al. Sideroblastic anemia. A diagnosis to consider in alcoholic patients. Postgrad Med 1992;92(7):147–50.

17. Simon SR, Branda RF, Tindle BF, et al. Copper deficiency and sideroblastic anemia associated with zinc ingestion. Am J Hematol 1988;28(3):181–3.

18. Beck EA, Ziegler G, Schmid R, et al. Reversible sideroblastic anemia caused by chloramphenicol. Acta Haematol 1967;38(1):1–10.

19. Willekens C, Dumezy F, Boyer T, et al. Linezolid induces ring sideroblasts. Haematologica 2013;98(11):e138–40.

20. Ponka P. Tissue-specific regulation of iron metabolism and heme synthesis: distinct control mechanisms in erythroid cells. Blood 1997;89(1):1–25.

21. Bewersdorf JP, Zeidan AM. Transforming growth factor (TGF)-beta pathway as a therapeutic target in lower risk myelodysplastic syndromes. Leukemia 2019; 33(6):1303–12.

22. Raza A, Gezer S, Mundle S, et al. Apoptosis in bone marrow biopsy samples involving stromal and hematopoietic cells in 50 patients with myelodysplastic syndromes. Blood 1995;86(1):268–76.

23. Thomas ML. Quality of life and psychosocial adjustment in patients with myelodysplastic syndromes. Leuk Res 1998;22(Suppl 1):S41–7.

24. Kornblith AB, Herndon JE 2nd, Silverman LR, et al. Impact of azacytidine on the quality of life of patients with myelodysplastic syndrome treated in a randomized phase III trial: a Cancer and Leukemia Group B study. J Clin Oncol 2002;20(10): 2441–52.

25. Hellstrom-Lindberg E, Gulbrandsen N, Lindberg G, et al. A validated decision model for treating the anaemia of myelodysplastic syndromes with erythropoietin + granulocyte colony-stimulating factor: significant effects on quality of life. Br J Haematol 2003;120(6):1037–46.

26. Park S, Greenberg P, Yucel A, et al. Clinical effectiveness and safety of erythropoietin-stimulating agents for the treatment of low- and intermediate-1-risk myelodysplastic syndrome: a systematic literature review. Br J Haematol 2019;184(2):134–60.

27. Greenberg PL, Sun Z, Miller KB, et al. Treatment of myelodysplastic syndrome patients with erythropoietin with or without granulocyte colony-stimulating factor: results of a prospective randomized phase 3 trial by the Eastern Cooperative Oncology Group (E1996). Blood 2009;114(12):2393–400.

28. Migdady Y, Barnard J, Al Ali N, et al. Clinical outcomes with ring sideroblasts and SF3B1 mutations in myelodysplastic syndromes: MDS clinical research consortium analysis. Clin Lymphoma Myeloma Leuk 2018;18(8):528–32.

29. Steensma DP. Myelodysplastic syndromes current treatment algorithm 2018. Blood Cancer J 2018;8(5):47.

30. Santini V. Clinical use of erythropoietic stimulating agents in myelodysplastic syndromes. Oncologist 2011;16(Suppl 3):35–42.

31. Cheson BD, Greenberg PL, Bennett JM, et al. Clinical application and proposal for modification of the International Working Group (IWG) response criteria in myelodysplasia. Blood 2006;108(2):419–25.

32. Fenaux P, Santini V, Spiriti MAA, et al. A phase 3 randomized, placebo-controlled study assessing the efficacy and safety of epoetin-alpha in anemic patients with low-risk MDS. Leukemia 2018;32(12):2648–58.

33. Ferrini PR, Grossi A, Vannucchi AM, et al. A randomized double-blind placebo-controlled study with subcutaneous recombinant human erythropoietin in patients with low-risk myelodysplastic syndromes. Br J Haematol 1998;103(4):1070–4.

34. Patton J, Reeves T, Wallace J. Effectiveness of darbepoetin alfa versus epoetin alfa in patients with chemotherapy-induced anemia treated in clinical practice. Oncologist 2004;9(4):451–8.

35. Platzbecker U, Symeonidis A, Oliva EN, et al. A phase 3 randomized placebo-controlled trial of darbepoetin alfa in patients with anemia and lower-risk myelodysplastic syndromes. Leukemia 2017;31(9):1944–50.

36. Hellstrom-Lindberg E. Efficacy of erythropoietin in the myelodysplastic syndromes: a meta-analysis of 205 patients from 17 studies. Br J Haematol 1995; 89(1):67–71.

37. Moyo V, Lefebvre P, Duh MS, et al. Erythropoiesis-stimulating agents in the treatment of anemia in myelodysplastic syndromes: a meta-analysis. Ann Hematol 2008;87(7):527–36.

38. Jadersten M, Montgomery SM, Dybedal I, et al. Long-term outcome of treatment of anemia in MDS with erythropoietin and G-CSF. Blood 2005;106(3):803–11.

39. Fink EC, Ebert BL. The novel mechanism of lenalidomide activity. Blood 2015; 126(21):2366–9.

40. Santini V, Almeida A, Giagounidis A, et al. Randomized phase III study of lenalidomide versus placebo in RBC transfusion-dependent patients with lower-risk

Non-del(5q) myelodysplastic syndromes and ineligible for or refractory to erythropoiesis-stimulating agents. J Clin Oncol 2016;34(25):2988–96.

41. Raza A, Reeves JA, Feldman EJ, et al. Phase 2 study of lenalidomide in transfusion-dependent, low-risk, and intermediate-1 risk myelodysplastic syndromes with karyotypes other than deletion 5q. Blood 2008;111(1):86–93.

42. Toma A, Kosmider O, Chevret S, et al. Lenalidomide with or without erythropoietin in transfusion-dependent erythropoiesis-stimulating agent-refractory lower-risk MDS without 5q deletion. Leukemia 2016;30(4):897–905.

43. List AF, Sun Z, Verma A, et al. Combined Treatment with Lenalidomide (LEN) and Epoetin Alfa (EA) is superior to lenalidomide alone in patients with Erythropoietin (Epo)-Refractory, Lower Risk (LR) non-deletion 5q [Del(5q)] Myelodysplastic Syndrome (MDS): results of the E2905 Intergroup Study-an ECOG-ACRIN Cancer Research Group Study, Grant CA180820, and the National Cancer Institute of the National Institutes of Health. Blood 2016;128(22):223.

44. Nicolosi M, Mudireddy M, Vallapureddy R, et al. Lenalidomide therapy in patients with myelodysplastic syndrome/myeloproliferative neoplasm with ring sideroblasts and thrombocytosis (MDS/MPN-RS-T). Am J Hematol 2018;93(1):E27–30.

45. Alshaban A, Padilla O, Philipovskiy A, et al. Lenalidomide induced durable remission in a patient with MDS/MPN-with ring sideroblasts and thrombocytosis with associated 5q- syndrome. Leuk Res Rep 2018;10:37–40.

46. Idossa D, Lasho TL, Finke CM, et al. Mutations and karyotype predict treatment response in myelodysplastic syndromes. Am J Hematol 2018;93(11):1420–6.

47. Brunner AM, Weng S, Cronin A, et al. Impact of lenalidomide use among non-transfusion dependent patients with myelodysplastic syndromes. Am J Hematol 2018;93(9):1119–26.

48. Platzbecker U, Germing U, Gotze KS, et al. Luspatercept for the treatment of anaemia in patients with lower-risk myelodysplastic syndromes (PACE-MDS): a multicentre, open-label phase 2 dose-finding study with long-term extension study. Lancet Oncol 2017;18(10):1338–47.

49. Carrancio S, Markovics J, Wong P, et al. An activin receptor IIA ligand trap promotes erythropoiesis resulting in a rapid induction of red blood cells and haemoglobin. Br J Haematol 2014;165(6):870–82.

50. Fenaux P, Platzbecker U, Mufti GJ, et al. The medalist trial: results of a phase 3, randomized, double-blind, placebo-controlled study of luspatercept to treat anemia in patients with very low-, low-, or intermediate-risk myelodysplastic syndromes (MDS) with ring sideroblasts (RS) who require red blood cell (RBC) transfusions. Blood 2018;132(Suppl 1):1.

51. Komrokji R, Garcia-Manero G, Ades L, et al. Sotatercept with long-term extension for the treatment of anaemia in patients with lower-risk myelodysplastic syndromes: a phase 2, dose-ranging trial. Lancet Haematol 2018;5(2):e63–72.

52. Tefferi A, Lasho TL, Begna KH, et al. A pilot study of the telomerase inhibitor imetelstat for myelofibrosis. N Engl J Med 2015;373(10):908–19.

53. Tefferi A, Al-Kali A, Begna KH, et al. Imetelstat therapy in refractory anemia with ring sideroblasts with or without thrombocytosis. Blood Cancer J 2016;6:e405.

54. Steensma DP, Platzbecker U, Van Eygen K, et al. Imetelstat treatment leads to durable transfusion independence (TI) in RBC transfusion-dependent (TD), non-del(5q) lower risk MDS relapsed/refractory to erythropoiesis-stimulating agent (ESA) who are lenalidomide (LEN) and HMA naive. Blood 2018;132(Suppl 1):463.

55. Seiler M, Yoshimi A, Darman R, et al. H3B-8800, an orally available small-molecule splicing modulator, induces lethality in spliceosome-mutant cancers. Nat Med 2018;24(4):497–504.

56. Colunga-Pedraza PR, Colunga-Pedraza JE, Garza-Ledezma MA, et al. Danazol as first-line therapy for myelodysplastic syndrome. Clin Lymphoma Myeloma Leuk 2018;18(2):e109–13.

57. Chan G, DiVenuti G, Miller K. Danazol for the treatment of thrombocytopenia in patients with myelodysplastic syndrome. Am J Hematol 2002;71(3):166–71.

58. Mittelman M, Platzbecker U, Afanasyev B, et al. Eltrombopag for advanced myelodysplastic syndromes or acute myeloid leukaemia and severe thrombocytopenia (ASPIRE): a randomised, placebo-controlled, phase 2 trial. Lancet Haematol 2018;5(1):e34–43.

59. Dickinson M, Cherif H, Fenaux P, et al. Azacitidine with or without eltrombopag for first-line treatment of intermediate- or high-risk MDS with thrombocytopenia. Blood 2018;132(25):2629–38.

60. Hoffbrand AV, Taher A, Cappellini MD. How I treat transfusional iron overload. Blood 2012;120(18):3657–69.

61. Shenoy N, Vallumsetla N, Rachmilewitz E, et al. Impact of iron overload and potential benefit from iron chelation in low-risk myelodysplastic syndrome. Blood 2014;124(6):873–81.

62. Angelucci E, Li J, Greenberg PL, et al. Safety and efficacy, including event-free survival, of deferasirox versus placebo in iron-overloaded patients with low- and Int-1-risk myelodysplastic syndromes (MDS): outcomes from the randomized, double-blind telesto study. Blood 2018;132(Suppl 1):234.

63. Greenberg PL, Stone RM, Al-Kali A, et al. Myelodysplastic syndromes, Version 2.2017, NCCN clinical practice guidelines in oncology. J Natl Compr Canc Netw 2017;15(1):60–87.

64. Malcovati L, Hellstrom-Lindberg E, Bowen D, et al. Diagnosis and treatment of primary myelodysplastic syndromes in adults: recommendations from the European LeukemiaNet. Blood 2013;122(17):2943–64.

65. Silverman LR, Demakos EP, Peterson BL, et al. Randomized controlled trial of azacitidine in patients with the myelodysplastic syndrome: a study of the cancer and leukemia group B. J Clin Oncol 2002;20(10):2429–40.

66. Thepot S, Ben Abdelali R, Chevret S, et al. A randomized phase II trial of azacitidine +/- epoetin-beta in lower-risk myelodysplastic syndromes resistant to erythropoietic stimulating agents. Haematologica 2016;101(8):918–25.

67. Garcia-Manero G, Jabbour E, Borthakur G, et al. Randomized open-label phase II study of decitabine in patients with low- or intermediate-risk myelodysplastic syndromes. J Clin Oncol 2013;31(20):2548–53.

68. Jabbour E, Short NJ, Montalban-Bravo G, et al. Randomized phase 2 study of low-dose decitabine vs low-dose azacitidine in lower-risk MDS and MDS/MPN. Blood 2017;130(13):1514–22.

69. Savona MR, Odenike O, Amrein PC, et al. An oral fixed-dose combination of decitabine and cedazuridine in myelodysplastic syndromes: a multicentre, open-label, dose-escalation, phase 1 study. Lancet Haematol 2019;6(4):e194–203.

70. Garcia-Manero G, Roboz G, Walsh K, et al. Guadecitabine (SGI-110) in patients with intermediate or high-risk myelodysplastic syndromes: phase 2 results from a multicentre, open-label, randomised, phase 1/2 trial. Lancet Haematol 2019;6(6):e317–27.

71. Stahl M, DeVeaux M, de Witte T, et al. The use of immunosuppressive therapy in MDS: clinical outcomes and their predictors in a large international patient cohort. Blood Adv 2018;2(14):1765–72.

72. Mangaonkar AA, Ferrer A, Pinto EVF, et al. Clinical applications and utility of a precision medicine approach for patients with unexplained cytopenias. Mayo Clin Proc 2019;94(9):1753–68.

73. Vairo FPE, Ferrer A, Cathcart-Rake E, et al. Novel germline missense DDX41 variant in a patient with an adult-onset myeloid neoplasm with excess blasts without dysplasia. Leuk Lymphoma 2019;60(5):1337–9.

74. Mangaonkar AA, Ferrer A, Pinto EVF, et al. Clinical correlates and treatment outcomes for patients with short telomere syndromes. Mayo Clin Proc 2018;93(7):834–9.

75. Mangaonkar AA, Patnaik MM. Short telomere syndromes in clinical practice: bridging bench and bedside. Mayo Clin Proc 2018;93(7):904–16.

76. Cutler CS, Lee SJ, Greenberg P, et al. A decision analysis of allogeneic bone marrow transplantation for the myelodysplastic syndromes: delayed transplantation for low-risk myelodysplasia is associated with improved outcome. Blood 2004;104(2):579–85.

77. Koreth J, Pidala J, Perez WS, et al. Role of reduced-intensity conditioning allogeneic hematopoietic stem-cell transplantation in older patients with de novo myelodysplastic syndromes: an international collaborative decision analysis. J Clin Oncol 2013;31(21):2662–70.

78. de Witte T, Bowen D, Robin M, et al. Allogeneic hematopoietic stem cell transplantation for MDS and CMML: recommendations from an international expert panel. Blood 2017;129(13):1753–62.

79. Broseus J, Florensa L, Zipperer E, et al. Clinical features and course of refractory anemia with ring sideroblasts associated with marked thrombocytosis. Haematologica 2012;97(7):1036–41.

80. Visconte V, Makishima H, Jankowska A, et al. SF3B1, a splicing factor is frequently mutated in refractory anemia with ring sideroblasts. Leukemia 2012;26(3):542–5.

81. Patnaik MM, Lasho TL, Finke CM, et al. Vascular events and risk factors for thrombosis in refractory anemia with ring sideroblasts and thrombocytosis. Leukemia 2016;30(11):2273–5.

82. Tefferi A, Vannucchi AM, Barbui T. Essential thrombocythemia treatment algorithm 2018. Blood Cancer J 2018;8(1):2.

83. Cazzola M, Malcovati L. Diagnosis and treatment of sideroblastic anemias: from defective heme synthesis to abnormal RNA splicing. Hematology Am Soc Hematol Educ Program 2015;2015:19–25.

84. DiNardo CD, Stein EM, de Botton S, et al. Durable remissions with ivosidenib in IDH1-mutated relapsed or refractory AML. N Engl J Med 2018;378(25):2386–98.

85. Stein EM, DiNardo CD, Fathi AT, et al. Molecular remission and response patterns in patients with mutant-IDH2 acute myeloid leukemia treated with enasidenib. Blood 2019;133(7):676–87.

86. DiNardo CD, Jabbour E, Ravandi F, et al. IDH1 and IDH2 mutations in myelodysplastic syndromes and role in disease progression. Leukemia 2016;30(4):980–4.

87. Visconte V, Kelly KR, Nawrocki ST, et al. Elevated basal autophagy in SF3B1 mutated myelodysplastic syndromes: relationship with survival outcomes and therapeutic implications. Blood 2015;126(23):1647.

Targeting *TP53* Mutations in Myelodysplastic Syndromes

Anthony M. Hunter, MD[a,b], David A. Sallman, MD[a,*]

KEYWORDS

- Myelodysplastic syndrome • *TP53* • Therapy-related myelodysplastic syndrome
- *TP53* mutant MDS

KEY POINTS

- The *TP53* gene is recurrently mutated in myelodysplastic syndromes and is associated with unique clinical and pathologic features.
- Demonstrating an unequivocal association with inferior outcomes, mutations in *TP53* play a critical role in prognostication and treatment selection.
- Hypomethylating agents remain the standard frontline treatment with allogeneic hematopoietic stem cell transplant an option in selected patients; however, long-term outcomes are poor.
- Novel agents are required to improve outcomes in *TP53*-mutated MDS and patients should be enrolled in clinical trials when available.

INTRODUCTION

Myelodysplastic syndromes (MDS) represent a group of clonal myeloid neoplasms with a high degree of variability in regards to their clinical phenotype, prognosis, and response to treatment. Current techniques in next-generation sequencing have allowed for large-scale analysis of the molecular underpinnings of the disease in an attempt to uncover biologic drivers of this diversity.[1–3] This has led to the discovery of an array of recurrently mutated genes involved in diverse cellular processes, such as DNA methylation, chromatin modification, signal transduction, transcriptional regulation, and RNA splicing.[1–8] Although the mechanisms by which these diverse pathways converge in the pathogenesis of MDS have not been fully elucidated, molecularly targeted therapies are under development and numerous studies have investigated the correlation of these mutations with clinical outcomes.[2,9–14] Although this work has implicated several genes as predictors of survival or response to

[a] Malignant Hematology, H. Lee Moffitt Cancer Center and Research Institute, GME office, 12902 USF Magnolia Drive, Tampa, FL 33612, USA; [b] University of South Florida, Morsani College of Medicine, 12901 Bruce B. Downs Blvd., Tampa, FL 33612, USA
* Corresponding author.
E-mail address: David.Sallman@moffitt.org

Hematol Oncol Clin N Am 34 (2020) 421–440
https://doi.org/10.1016/j.hoc.2019.11.004
0889-8588/20/© 2019 Elsevier Inc. All rights reserved.

hemonc.theclinics.com

therapy, mutations in *TP53* carry perhaps the greatest importance because of their unequivocal association with dismal outcomes in patients with MDS.

Labeled the "guardian of the genome" because of its essential tumor suppressor functionality, the *TP53* gene, located on chromosome 17p13.1, is mutated in nearly half of all tumors making it the most widely mutated gene in human malignancy.[15–17] Its protein product, p53, functions as a transcription factor that is tightly regulated by several mechanisms including post-translational modifications and interaction with the negative regulator, MDM2.[18–20] The protein contains several functional domains including an N-terminal transactivation domain, a proline-rich SH3 domain, a tetramerization domain, the C-terminal regulatory domain, and a vital DNA-binding domain.[20,21] These domains are critical in protein activation in response to cellular stresses, such as DNA damage, oncogene activation, and ribonucleotide depletion, and carrying out the transcriptional regulation of p53 target genes, which are involved in a variety of cellular processes including differentiation, DNA repair, cell cycle arrest, and initiation of apoptosis.[16,18,22]

The negative prognostic impact of *TP53* mutations observed in not only MDS, but a variety of malignancies, is supported by its crucial role in facilitating the cellular apoptotic response to DNA damaging agents, such as cytotoxic chemotherapy.[23–25] Mutant *TP53* has been shown to confer to cancer cells intrinsic resistance to common antineoplastic agents.[26,27] This underscores the importance of identifying *TP53* mutations when developing personalized treatment plans, and the need to develop agents with novel pharmacologic activity that does not rely on endogenous wild-type p53 function. In this review we discuss the impact of *TP53* mutations in the treatment of MDS and highlight therapies currently under investigation with a potential role in this challenging patient cohort.

SPECTRUM AND CLINICAL CHARACTERISTICS OF *TP53* MUTATIONS IN MYELODYSPLASTIC SYNDROMES

Mutations in *TP53* are observed in up to 20% of patients with MDS, considerably lower than that observed in other malignancies.[1,2,28] Most mutations are missense mutations, although insertion/deletions, splice-site mutations, and nonsense mutations are observed at lower frequencies.[29,30] Although mutations are observed throughout the entirety of the gene, up to 90% occur in the DNA binding domain with a penchant for arginine residues, including codons 248 and 273.[30,31] Although mutations in other functional domains, including gain-of-function mutations, have distinctive biologic activity, the clinical relevance of these is not defined.[32,33] Although *TP53* mutations are readily captured by current next-generation sequencing panels, increased levels of p53 protein detected by immunohistochemical techniques have also been shown to accurately correlate with mutation status and may be used as a surrogate in settings where sequencing is not available.[30,34]

TP53 mutated patients have a lower than expected frequency of concurrent mutations in several common MDS-associated genes including ASXL1, RUNX1, and the spliceosome genes.[30,31,35] Up to 70% have no additional somatic mutations in contrast to wild-type patients who have a median of approximately three mutated genes.[2,31,35,36] The median variant allele frequency (VAF) is among the highest of recurrently mutated genes in MDS with an elevated VAF predicting for an increased probability of complex karyotype and inferior survival.[35,37] *TP53* mutations correlate strongly with complex and monosomal karyotypes, particularly those with loss of 5/5q, 7/7q, or 17/17p, occurring in 50% to 80% of such cases.[28,30,31,35] Although complex karyotype and *TP53* mutations are independent predictors of survival, *TP53* mutation status remained the strongest predictor of survival in multivariate analyses of the largest evaluated cohort of complex karyotype patients with MDS.[35] Additionally, *TP53* mutations are observed in 10% to 20% of cases of MDS with isolated del(5q) and are associated with inferior survival and an increased risk of progression in this traditionally lower-risk subtype.[30,38–40]

In comparison with wild-type patients, *TP53* mutations are associated with older age, lower white blood cell count, lower platelet count, higher bone marrow blast percentage, and higher-risk disease by IPSS-R classification.[28,31,35] Based on these high risk features, many clinical trials and prognostic cohorts are significantly enriched in *TP53* mutant patients whereby this molecular cohort frequently represents 20% of patients.[31,41,42] Additionally, *TP53* mutations are enriched in cases of therapy-related MDS, occurring in 30% to 40% of such cases.[43–45] *TP53* mutations are strong independent predictors for inferior overall survival (OS) and risk of transformation to acute myeloid leukemia (AML).[13,14,28] Although they are not yet incorporated into current risk stratification systems, *TP53* mutations represent perhaps the single greatest prognostic determinant in MDS and thus identification is of the utmost importance in prognostication and treatment selection, because it is detailed in this review.

EFFICACY OF STANDARD THERAPEUTIC APPROACHES IN *TP53*-MUTATED MYELODYSPLASTIC SYNDROMES
Hypomethylating Agents

To date, two hypomethylating agents (HMAs) have been approved for the treatment of MDS in the United States: azacytidine and decitabine. Both function as nucleoside analogues that incorporate into DNA, with azacytidine also demonstrating the ability to incorporate into RNA. Although multiple cellular effects are observed, their predominant mechanism is thought to be related to depletion of DNA methyltransferases with resultant global DNA hypomethylation, and induction of DNA damage.[46,47]

The approval of azacytidine in MDS was based on the phase 3 AZA-001 trial that demonstrated a significant improvement in median OS in patients treated with azacytidine (24.5 months) compared with those randomized to conventional care regimens (15 months).[48] Several clinical trials have also demonstrated clinical activity with decitabine in MDS, although a survival advantage has not been clearly demonstrated.[49–51] As a result of this work, HMAs have become the standard frontline treatment option in patients with higher-risk MDS, regardless of World Health Organization subtype or FAB classification.

Preclinical study has demonstrated that *TP53* mutations increase the sensitivity of cells to HMA treatment, making this a potentially desirable treatment option in *TP53*-mutated MDS.[52,53] A single-center prospective study using a 10-day regimen of decitabine in AML and patients with MDS demonstrated that *TP53* mutations were associated with improved response rates and that the negative prognostic impact of *TP53* mutations was not observed in the total cohort treated with decitabine.[54] However, although the rate of blast clearance was significantly improved (100% in *TP53*-mutated vs 41% in wild-type patients), the rate of complete response (CR) was not (19%, compared with 14% in wild-type patients; $P = .73$) and a trend toward inferior survival was observed in the MDS subgroup ($P = .08$). Although other studies have suggested improved response rates to HMA,[55] several clinical studies have evaluated molecular predictors of outcomes with HMA therapy and have not shown a significant difference in response rates between *TP53*-mutated and wild-type patients.[12,13,30,31,56] Similarly, *TP53* mutations were associated with a shorter duration of response to HMA and remained predictive of inferior OS in these studies.

In contrast to other recurrent somatic mutations seen in MDS, HMA therapy does result in a reduction in *TP53* mutational burden in treated patients, which is rarely seen with other genes.[54,56] However, despite this reduction, the *TP53* clone remains detectable at low levels in all cases. Recently presented work demonstrated that *TP53* clonal clearance (defined as VAF <5%) was associated with an improvement in OS in HMA-treated patients, regardless of response, suggesting a role for sequential molecular testing during therapy and identifying a potentially important prognostic determinant in this subgroup.[41]

Although current data suggest that HMAs do not completely abrogate the poor outcomes seen in *TP53*-mutated MDS, clinical benefit is observed and comparison of HMAs with other therapies in this group are lacking. As such, they remain the standard frontline treatment option for patients in whom a clinical trial is not an option. Although decitabine has been preferred in *TP53* mutant patients by some centers, recently presented work demonstrated no significant difference in outcomes with azacytidine compared with decitabine and an additional study has suggested no difference in efficacy between 5-day and 10-day regimens of decitabine in patients with AML.[57,58]

Lenalidomide

MDS with isolated del(5q) is recognized as a distinct subgroup by the World Health Organization and is characterized by unique clinicobiologic features including a profound hypoplastic anemia.[59] The immunomodulatory agent lenalidomide has demonstrated the ability to reverse transfusion dependence and produce cytogenetic remissions in patients with del(5q) leading to its approval in this setting.[60] Preclinical studies have demonstrated that the pathophysiology of MDS with del(5q) involves p53 activation in erythroid precursors and that downstream activity of lenalidomide reverses this by stabilizing MDM2 and promoting p53 degradation, with *TP53* mutations thus conferring potential resistance.[61–65] Clinical studies have evaluated small numbers of patients, but have variably shown decreased responses with shortened OS, emergence and/or expansion of *TP53* mutant clones, and an increased risk of AML transformation compared with wild-type patients.[39,66–68] Although response rates are still reasonably high, consideration should be given to alternative therapies, such as HMA, particularly in younger patients that are transplant eligible, given these concerns. Moreover, a Nordic MDS group trial evaluating high-risk patients with MDS with a karyotype harboring del(5q), a cohort expected to be enriched in *TP53* mutations, identified no benefit with the addition of lenalidomide to azacytidine (overall response rate, 36% for azacytidine alone vs 28% for combination; median OS 14 months with azacytidine vs 10 months with combination) providing clear evidence against the use of this combination.[69]

Allogeneic Hematopoietic Stem Cell Transplant

Standard treatment options in MDS target control of the disease by improving cytopenias; relieving symptoms; delaying progression to AML; and, in the case of azacytidine, extending survival. Yet, no current treatment possesses curative potential outside of an allogeneic hematopoietic stem cell transplant (allo-HSCT). Although typically not indicated in lower-risk patients, who may do well for years, higher-risk patients with MDS have significant morbidity and mortality and thus allo-HSCT should be considered in all patients who are candidates.[70] Although this results in long-term survival in up to 30% to 50% of patients with MDS, the use of allo-HSCT in *TP53*-mutated patients has been debated because of less optimistic outcomes in this molecular subgroup.[71–74]

An array of studies have evaluated molecular and clinical predictors of outcomes in patients with MDS undergoing allo-HSCT. Although individual studies have identified several genes that predict for inferior outcomes, *TP53* mutations are the most notable because they have been consistently identified as the strongest predictor among all clinical and molecular variables analyzed and were the only gene reliably identified across all studies.[9,14,75,76] The 2- to 4-year survival rates among *TP53*-mutated patients in these studies range from 10% to 20%, with some reporting no long-term survivors, and mortality largely resulting from early relapse without a significant increase in transplant-related mortality.

Although these dismal outcomes have led to some debating the appropriateness of allo-HSCT in *TP53*-mutated patients with MDS, long-term survival is observed in a subset of patients that could not otherwise be achieved and thus allo-HSCT should still be pursued in the appropriate context.[77] Careful patient selection, the use of optimal bridging therapies in the pretransplant setting, and post-transplant maintenance therapies have the potential to optimize outcomes in this cohort, although further study is required. The use of HMA as a bridge to allo-HSCT has been proposed as a method to attenuate the poor outcomes observed in this group, with Welch and colleagues[54] demonstrating that *TP53* mutations did not negatively impact survival after allo-HSCT following a 10-day decitabine regimen. However, *TP53* mutations remained a strong negative predictor of survival in post hoc analysis from the prospective BMT-AZA trial, with response to azacytidine treatment also an important predictor.[56] Our group has identified a survival benefit for allo-HSCT in patients with clonal clearance after HMA therapy with no benefit observed in patients with a persistent clone, suggesting that sequential monitoring of *TP53* mutational burden during HMA therapy may prove a useful tool in selecting patients for transplant.[41] Furthermore, detection of at least one somatic mutation with a VAF greater than or equal to 0.5% at 30 days post allo-HSCT has been shown to be predictive of inferior progression-free survival in patients with MDS, with 75% of *TP53* mutations remaining detectable at this time point.[78] Notably, among those patients with a detectable mutation after allo-HSCT, the use of a reduced intensity conditioning regimen was associated with inferior progression-free survival compared with those who had received myeloablative conditioning, underscoring the role of conditioning therapy in outcomes.

Post-transplant HMA maintenance therapy has also been evaluated, with initial single-arm studies demonstrating feasibility and the potential to reduce relapse rates.[79–81] This approach was subsequently evaluated in a randomized trial, which did not demonstrate an improvement in relapse-free survival, although there were significant limitations to the study and *TP53*-specific outcomes were not presented.[82] Histone deacetylase (HDAC) inhibitors have also been tested in this setting and may be appealing because of their effect on mutant p53.[83] A single arm trial has reported favorable outcomes compared with historical control subjects, although insufficient data exist at this time to recommend this approach in routine practice.[84]

EMERGING THERAPIES IN *TP53* MUTANT MYELODYSPLASTIC SYNDROMES

In light of the generally poor outcomes observed with standard therapies and inherent resistance that *TP53* mutations confer against traditional cytotoxic agents, therapies with novel mechanisms are required to raise the bar in this challenging subgroup. As such, all patients should be considered for treatment on clinical trial protocols evaluating novel agents. Although a variety of therapies are currently under investigation, they are divided into two groups: targeted therapies and immunotherapies (summarized in **Table 1**).

Table 1
Therapies currently under investigation in MDS with potential in *TP53* mutated disease

Therapeutic Class	Agent	Mechanism of Action	Studied Population	Results Reported to Date	Phase of Development	Ongoing Trials in MDS (NCT No.)	Reference
Bcl-2 inhibitor	Venetoclax[a]	Inhibits the antiapoptotic protein Bcl-2	Frontline treatment in elderly or medically unfit patients with AML; in combination with HMA or LDAC	Overall: CR/CRi in 67%, mOS of 17.5 mo *TP53* mutant (n = 36) Outcomes: CR/CRi in 47%, mOS of 7.2 mo	Accelerated FDA approval for frontline treatment of AML (11/21/18)	NCT02942290, NCT02966782	Vo et al,[91] 2012
NEDD8 inhibitor	Pevonedistat[a]	NEDD8 activating enzyme inhibitor	Frontline treatment in patients with AML unfit for chemotherapy; in combination with AZA	ORR of 50% (80% in *TP53*-mutated cases; n = 5)	Phase 3	NCT03268954, NCT03459859, NCT03772925	Malhab et al,[97] 2016
HDAC inhibitors	Multiple agents have been studied	Epigenetic regulation and mutant p53 degradation	De novo or R/R AML and high-risk MDS (as combination therapy); post-allo-HSCT maintenance	CR in ~15%–40% in combination with HMA (no clear improvement over HMA monotherapy)	Phase 3	NCT03772925, NCT02936752	Li et al,[102] 2011; Dennis et al,[103] 2016; Nishioka et al,[104] 2011; Craddock et al, 2017[105]
Statins	Atorvastatin	HMG-CoA reductase inhibitor; degrades mutant p53	*TP53* mutant relapsed AML and solid tumors	Not reported	Pilot trial	NCT03560882	No results reported from clinical study
TP53 reactivators	APR-246[a]	Restores WT *TP53* conformation and function	*TP53* mutated MDS, in combination with AZA	CR in 82% (9/11), mOS and mPFS NR (all *TP53* mutant)	Phase 3	NCT03745716, NCT03931291	Ali et al,[118] 2011

				Results	Phase	NCT numbers	References
Checkpoint inhibitors	Nivolumab	Anti-PD-1 monoclonal antibody	Frontline or prior HMA therapy, alone or in combination with HMA ± ipilimumab	With HMA: ORR 75% Alone: ORR 13% Aza + Nivo + Ipi: ORR 50% frontline, 29% in HMA failure	Phase 2	NCT02530463, NCT03600155, NCT03417154, NCT04044209, NCT02397720	Orskov et al,[126] 2015; Davids et al,[127] 2016
	Ipilimumab	Anti-CTLA-4 monoclonal antibody	Frontline or prior HMA therapy, alone or in combination with HMA ± nivolumab; relapse post-allo-HSCT	With HMA: ORR 71% Alone: ORR 35% Relapse post-allo-HSCT: CR in 5/22 (all myeloid diseases)	Phase 2	NCT02530463, NCT03600155, NCT02890329	Zajac et al,[124] 2016; Orskov et al,[126] 2015; Davids et al,[127] 2016
	Hu5F9-G4	Anti-CD47 monoclonal antibody (macrophage immune checkpoint)	R/R AML and MDS, frontline AML (unfit for induction therapy) and high-risk MDS	CR in 53% of untreated patients; 50% of responders MRD-negative; HI in 80% of MDS patients	Phase 1b	NCT03248479	Jaiswal et al,[132] 2009
Bispecific antibodies	Flotetuzumab (MGD006)	CD123xCD3 DART antibody	R/R AML and high-risk MDS	ORR of 43% in initial cohort	Phase 2	NCT02152956, NCT03739606	Sallman et al,[135] 2019; Hoseini & Cheung,[136] 2017
CAR T-cell therapy	CYAD-01	NKG2D receptor expressing CAR T cells	R/R AML and MDS	CRi/CRh in 42% (3/7 patients) treated with multiple infusions, MDS results not reported	Phase 1/2	NCT03018405, NCT03466320	Ravandi et al,[140] 2018
	ICG144	CLL1-CD33 compound CAR T cells	R/R high-risk myeloid neoplasms	CR in 2 patients reported (both AML)	Phase 1	NCT03795779	Sallman et al,[143] 2018

Abbreviations: AZA, azacytidine; Bcl-2, B-cell lymphoma 2; CAR, chimeric antigen receptor; CRh, complete response with partial hematologic recovery; CRi, complete response with incomplete hematologic recovery; DART, dual-affinity retargeting; FDA, food and drug administration; HMG-CoA, 3-hydroxy-3-methylglutaryl coenzyme A; Ipi, ipilimumab; LDAC, low-dose cytarabine; mOS, median overall survival; mPFS, median progression-free survival; MRD, minimal residual disease; Nivo, nivolumab; NKG2D, Natural Killer Group 2D; NR, not reached; ORR, overall response rate; R/R, relapsed and/or refractory; WT, wild type.
^a Clinical therapeutics where mutant *TP53* specific responses and/or outcomes have been reported.

Targeted Therapies

Targeted therapies can affect mutant p53 via a variety of mechanisms including influencing integrated or downstream pathways, degrading the mutant protein, or restoring wild-type p53 function. TP53 is involved in an array of cellular pathways and thus interacts with and relies on the function a variety of additional proteins.[16] This gives rise to numerous potential targets that, when inhibited, may result in synthetic lethality in TP53-mutated cells. Preclinical work has indeed identified several such pathways including several kinase signaling pathways and regulators of the G2/M checkpoint.[29,85–87] Although the clinical utility of this approach is unknown at this time, further study is warranted because exploiting synthetic lethality has proven efficacious in other malignancies as evidenced by the use of PARP inhibitors in BRCA-mutated cancers.[88]

A critical cellular function of p53 is the induction of apoptosis, of which the antiapoptotic protein Bcl-2 is also a crucial regulator. Investigations have identified critical interactions between p53 and Bcl-2, with missense mutations within the TP53 DNA binding domain blocking complex formation and resulting in decreased apoptotic activity.[89,90] Bcl-2 has also been shown to have a role in the survival of leukemic blasts, with preclinical study identifying it as a promising therapeutic target.[91–93] This has led to clinical study of the Bcl-2 inhibitor venetoclax in combination with HMA, with a large phase 1b trial in patients with AML deemed unfit for induction chemotherapy demonstrating promising outcomes and leading to its recent approval in this setting.[42] However, subgroup analysis identified that TP53 mutations, found in 25% of evaluated patients, were associated with decreased response rates and inferior OS compared with the total cohort, raising the question if this combination is improving outcomes in TP53-mutated patients. In this regard, recent elegant investigations have highlighted that TP53 mutation drives venetoclax resistance by protecting cells from mitochondrial stress leading to impaired induction of apoptosis.[94] The authors showed in their TP53 knockout model that mutant cells acquired sensitivity to selective tyrosine receptor kinase inhibitors offering rationale for future drug combinations. Further clinical study of venetoclax in higher-risk patients with MDS is currently ongoing (NCT02942290, NCT02966782).

An additional agent that has recently shown promise in combination with HMA is the NEDD8-activating enzyme inhibitor, pevonedistat. The NEDD8 pathway is involved in the ubiquitin-proteasome system with addition of the ubiquitin-like protein NEDD8 required for activity of the Cullin-RING E3 ubiquitin ligase family, which directs protein degradation via the proteasome. This pathway has been shown to modulate the activity of p53, with resultant inhibition of p53 via Mdm2-dependent NEDDylation, and TP53 mutant cells have displayed increased sensitivity to NEDD8-activating enzyme inhibition.[95–98] Preclinical activity has demonstrated synergy with HMAs leading to a phase 1 study of pevonedistat in combination with HMA in patients with AML.[99] The combination resulted in an overall response rate of 50% with responses observed in 80% of TP53-mutated patients (n = 5), although sample size was limited.[100]

Mutant p53 protein demonstrates increased stability compared with wild-type p53 resulting in cellular accumulation and potential gain-of-function activity. Increasing degradation of mutant p53 protein has been hypothesized as a treatment strategy to directly target TP53-mutated cancer cells.[101] The HSP90 chaperone machinery and its activator, HDAC6, have been shown to play an integral role and have been suggested as potential targets.[102] HSP90 inhibitors, including ganetespib, have indeed demonstrated the ability to increase mutant p53 degradation; however, a randomized trial in AML did not demonstrate efficacy.[103] HDAC inhibitors have also shown the ability to destabilize mutant p53 protein and promising preclinical activity in *TP53*-mutated cells has been reported.[83,104] This has provided the rationale for several trials investigating HDAC inhibitors in the treatment of myeloid malignancies, alone or in combination; however, no significant benefit has been observed to date.[105–108] Yet, clinical studies remain ongoing because early drug discontinuation as a result of toxicity and pleiotropic effects of the studied agents may have contributed to these results with newer, more selective HDAC inhibitors a potential remedy.[109,110]

The statins are a widely used class of lipid-lowering medications that function by inhibiting 3-hydroxy-3-methylglutaryl coenzyme A reductase, the rate-limiting enzyme in the mevalonate pathway. Recent investigations have identified that tumors lacking p53 are vulnerable to inhibition of the mevalonate pathway, representing a potential novel therapeutic target.[111] Furthermore, statins are capable of inducing degradation of mutant p53, suppress the growth of *TP53*-mutated cancer cells, and display synergism with chemotherapeutic agents.[112–114] This provides rationale for statins as a novel component of combination therapies in *TP53*-mutated malignancies.

Finally, restoring wild-type p53 conformation and activity presents a promising therapeutic approach given the potential to target the unique biology of the disease and selectively act on malignant cells. Screens have identified a variety of compounds that are able to achieve reactivation of p53 activity, some of which target only specific *TP53* point mutations.[29] Although most have only been explored in preclinical models, APR-246, a methylated PRIMA-1 analogue, has now reached phase 3 study in *TP53*-mutated MDS and represents the most promising agent to date.

APR-246 is a small molecule that is spontaneously degraded into the active species, methylene quinuclidinone, which is able to covalently bond to cysteine residues in p53 thereby producing thermodynamic stabilization of the protein and shifting equilibrium toward the wild-type p53 conformation.[115] Indeed, this agent has been shown to restore wild-type p53 activity resulting in selective apoptosis of *TP53*-mutated cells and displaying synergism with several cytotoxic agents in leukemic cell lines.[116–118] Clinical activity in humans was first documented in two phase 1 trials using single agent APR-246, demonstrating promising activity in *TP53*-mutated myeloid malignancies.[119,120] This has led to further clinical study of APR-246 in combination with azacytidine in *TP53*-mutated MDS and AML. Preliminary data from a phase 1 b/2 study demonstrated that this combination regimen is tolerable and highly efficacious, with 82% of patients achieving CR and exhibiting deep molecular remissions.[121] The drug was subsequently granted fast track and orphan drug designations by the Food and Drug Administration and a multicenter phase 3 study is ongoing (NCT03745716).

Immunotherapies

Since the initial approval of the anti-CD20 monoclonal antibody rituximab in 1997, the use of immunotherapeutic agents in oncology has exploded. Encompassing a broad array of agents, immunotherapies use a variety of mechanisms that converge on the ability to exploit the intrinsic function of the host immune system to recognize and eliminate cells that have undergone malignant transformation. Although the use of immunotherapies in the treatment of myeloid malignancies has lagged, it is an approach that holds particular promise in *TP53*-mutated malignancies given the lack of reliance on p53-dependent apoptosis, in contrast to cytotoxic agents. It is currently an area of active clinical study in myeloid malignancies with monoclonal antibodies, immune checkpoint inhibitors, bispecific antibodies, and cellular therapies all currently under investigation.

Given the innate ability of the immune system to eliminate malignant cells, it is rationalized that any established cancer has developed the means to evade this function and a variety of such mechanisms have now been discovered. Perhaps the most widely studied to date are the "immune checkpoints," with inhibitory checkpoints, such as PD-1 and CTLA-4, able to suppress T-cell-mediated destruction of malignant cells. This has led to the development of checkpoint inhibitors, which are now approved for the treatment of a variety of malignancies.

Inhibitory checkpoints, including PD-1, have been shown to play a role in the pathogenesis of myeloid malignancies with studies documenting their presence on leukemic blasts and marrow infiltrating T-cells.[122,123] Further upregulation of these signals has been demonstrated in patients with *TP53* mutations in comparison with wild-type patients making checkpoint inhibition an intriguing therapy in *TP53*-mutated cases.[122,124,125] Treatment with HMAs has been shown to lead to upregulation of these signals suggesting a possible resistance mechanism to HMA and providing rationale for combination therapy.[123,126] This evidence has led to the clinical study of checkpoint inhibitors in myeloid malignancies in several settings. The first such study to be published evaluated the use of the CTLA-4 inhibitor, ipilimumab, in patients with relapsed hematologic malignancies following allo-HSCT with most responses seen in myeloid malignancies.[127] Results of a phase 2 study using the PD-1 inhibitor, nivolumab, in combination with azacytidine in relapsed/refractory AML have also been published demonstrating tolerability and efficacy (overall response rate, 33%), with *TP53* mutations not predicting for inferior outcomes.[128] Several trials of checkpoint inhibitors alone and/or in combination with HMA in patients with MDS are ongoing and preliminary data have been reported.[129,130] Acceptable toxicities have been observed with clinical activity higher in HMA/checkpoint combination therapy (overall response rate as high as 75% with azacitidine + nivolumab) compared with checkpoint therapy alone, although results of subgroup analysis in *TP53*-mutated patients have not been reported.

CD47 is a member of the immunoglobulin superfamily, which acts as a critical anti-phagocytic signal via binding to SIRPα on macrophages, playing an important role in the homeostatic clearance of aged or damaged cells and functioning as a "macrophage immune checkpoint."[131] Importantly, CD47 is upregulated by several cancers, including leukemic stem cells, allowing it to evade immune surveillance by conveying a "don't eat me" signal to phagocytic cells and has thus been identified as a potential therapeutic target.[132,133] A monoclonal antibody, Hu5F9-G4, targeting CD47 has now been developed with preclinical data demonstrating synergism with azacitidine, resulting in enhanced phagocytosis of AML blasts.[134] This has led to a phase 1b study testing this combination in patients with MDS and AML. Preliminary data have been reported demonstrating tolerability and promising activity, with a CR rate of 53% in treatment-naive patients and MRD negativity observed in 50% of responders.[135]

Finally, bispecific antibodies and cellular therapies, such as chimeric antigen receptor (CAR) T-cell therapy, are novel approaches that have greatly advanced the treatment of lymphoid malignancies in the past several years. However, their use in myeloid malignancies has been more challenging, in part because of difficulty in identifying candidate target antigens. In comparison with B-cell lymphoid malignancies, antigens in myeloid lineage malignancies are more heterogenous and less restricted, raising concerns for increased toxicity, such as hematopoietic cell aplasia (analogous to the B-cell aplasia seen with CD-19 CAR T-cell therapy). However, several potential targets have been identified and are under investigation in MDS and AML, including CD33, CD123, FLT3, CLL-1, and NKG2D.[136,137]

Although still in early phase clinical study, preliminary data have been presented using bispecific antibodies in MDS and AML. Flotetuzumab, a CD123xCD3 antibody, was studied in a population of relapsed/refractory AML and high-risk patients with

MDS with an overall response rate of 22% and cytokine release syndrome the most frequently observed toxicity (grade 3 in 13%).[138,139] Clinical activity and tolerability were also documented in a phase 1 trial evaluating the CD33xCD3 antibody, AMG 330, in a population of relapsed/refractory patients with AML.[140] No molecular subgroup analysis has been reported in these studies.

Several CAR T-cell products are currently under investigation, although initial studies are largely evaluating their use in patients with AML. The first documented objective response to CAR T-cell therapy in a patient with a myeloid malignancy was with the NKG2D receptor construct, CYAD-01.[141] Two phase 1 trials have been reported with this same construct demonstrating clinical activity, although only with the use of multiple cellular administrations.[142,143] Antileukemic activity has also been observed with CAR T-cell constructs targeting CD123 and CD33, and a compound CAR product targeting CLL1-CD33.[144–147] Although these preliminary data are intriguing, particularly given the efficacy of these approaches in advanced lymphoid malignancies, only a small number of patients have been treated to date and further study is required.

SUMMARY

Current next-generation sequencing technologies have allowed for the discovery of the recurrent somatic mutations that underlie MDS biology, with genes from a variety of molecular pathways now identified. Although many of these genes have been implicated in prognostication and treatment selection, mutations in the critical tumor suppressor gene, *TP53*, are the most critical. Representing a distinct genetic ontogeny, *TP53* mutations are associated with dismal outcomes in MDS, with *TP53*-mutated MDS and AML likely representing a uniform disease. Outcomes with traditional cytotoxic therapies are poor because of their reliance on endogenous p53 activity, with mutations conferring intrinsic resistance to such agents. Although activity with traditional therapies, such as HMA, lenalidomide, and allo-HSCT is observed in patients with MDS, outcomes are inferior and novel therapies are required in this challenging molecular subgroup. Agents that directly target the mutant p53 protein and immunotherapeutic approaches are strategies that hold particular promise in the disease, although further clinical study is required.

DISCLOSURE

A.M. Hunter: Nothing to disclose.
David Sallman: Research Funding from Celgene and Jazz.

REFERENCES

1. Papaemmanuil E, Gerstung M, Malcovati L, et al. Clinical and biological implications of driver mutations in myelodysplastic syndromes. Blood 2013;122(22):3616–27 [quiz: 3699].
2. Haferlach T, Nagata Y, Grossmann V, et al. Landscape of genetic lesions in 944 patients with myelodysplastic syndromes. Leukemia 2014;28(2):241–7.
3. Makishima H, Yoshizato T, Yoshida K, et al. Dynamics of clonal evolution in myelodysplastic syndromes. Nat Genet 2017;49(2):204–12.
4. Langemeijer SM, Kuiper RP, Berends M, et al. Acquired mutations in TET2 are common in myelodysplastic syndromes. Nat Genet 2009;41(7):838–42.
5. Walter MJ, Ding L, Shen D, et al. Recurrent DNMT3A mutations in patients with myelodysplastic syndromes. Leukemia 2011;25(7):1153–8.

6. Yoshida K, Sanada M, Shiraishi Y, et al. Frequent pathway mutations of splicing machinery in myelodysplasia. Nature 2011;478(7367):64–9.

7. Boultwood J, Perry J, Pellagatti A, et al. Frequent mutation of the polycomb-associated gene ASXL1 in the myelodysplastic syndromes and in acute myeloid leukemia. Leukemia 2010;24(5):1062–5.

8. Papaemmanuil E, Cazzola M, Boultwood J, et al. Somatic SF3B1 mutation in myelodysplasia with ring sideroblasts. N Engl J Med 2011;365(15):1384–95.

9. Bejar R, Stevenson KE, Caughey B, et al. Somatic mutations predict poor outcome in patients with myelodysplastic syndrome after hematopoietic stem-cell transplantation. J Clin Oncol 2014;32(25):2691–8.

10. Kennedy JA, Ebert BL. Clinical implications of genetic mutations in myelodysplastic syndrome. J Clin Oncol 2017;35(9):968–74.

11. Traina F, Visconte V, Elson P, et al. Impact of molecular mutations on treatment response to DNMT inhibitors in myelodysplasia and related neoplasms. Leukemia 2014;28(1):78–87.

12. Bejar R, Lord A, Stevenson K, et al. TET2 mutations predict response to hypomethylating agents in myelodysplastic syndrome patients. Blood 2014;124(17):2705–12.

13. Bally C, Ades L, Renneville A, et al. Prognostic value of TP53 gene mutations in myelodysplastic syndromes and acute myeloid leukemia treated with azacitidine. Leuk Res 2014;38(7):751–5.

14. Lindsley RC, Saber W, Mar BG, et al. Prognostic mutations in myelodysplastic syndrome after stem-cell transplantation. N Engl J Med 2017;376(6):536–47.

15. Vogelstein B, Lane D, Levine AJ. Surfing the p53 network. Nature 2000;408(6810):307–10.

16. Vousden KH, Lu X. Live or let die: the cell's response to p53. Nat Rev Cancer 2002;2(8):594–604.

17. Lane DP. Cancer. p53, guardian of the genome. Nature 1992;358(6381):15–6.

18. Levine AJ. p53, the cellular gatekeeper for growth and division. Cell 1997;88(3):323–31.

19. Oren M. Regulation of the p53 tumor suppressor protein. J Biol Chem 1999;274(51):36031–4.

20. Bode AM, Dong Z. Post-translational modification of p53 in tumorigenesis. Nat Rev Cancer 2004;4(10):793–805.

21. Harms KL, Chen X. The functional domains in p53 family proteins exhibit both common and distinct properties. Cell Death Differ 2006;13(6):890–7.

22. Harris SL, Levine AJ. The p53 pathway: positive and negative feedback loops. Oncogene 2005;24(17):2899–908.

23. Eliopoulos AG, Kerr DJ, Herod J, et al. The control of apoptosis and drug resistance in ovarian cancer: influence of p53 and Bcl-2. Oncogene 1995;11(7):1217–28.

24. Hamada M, Fujiwara T, Hizuta A, et al. The p53 gene is a potent determinant of chemosensitivity and radiosensitivity in gastric and colorectal cancers. J Cancer Res Clin Oncol 1996;122(6):360–5.

25. Fujiwara T, Grimm EA, Mukhopadhyay T, et al. Induction of chemosensitivity in human lung cancer cells in vivo by adenovirus-mediated transfer of the wild-type p53 gene. Cancer Res 1994;54(9):2287–91.

26. Lowe SW, Bodis S, McClatchey A, et al. p53 status and the efficacy of cancer therapy in vivo. Science 1994;266(5186):807–10.

27. Li R, Sutphin PD, Schwartz D, et al. Mutant p53 protein expression interferes with p53-independent apoptotic pathways. Oncogene 1998;16(25):3269–77.

28. Bejar R, Stevenson K, Abdel-Wahab O, et al. Clinical effect of point mutations in myelodysplastic syndromes. N Engl J Med 2011;364(26):2496–506.

29. Zhao D, Tahaney WM, Mazumdar A, et al. Molecularly targeted therapies for p53-mutant cancers. Cell Mol Life Sci 2017;74(22):4171–87.

30. Kulasekararaj AG, Smith AE, Mian SA, et al. TP53 mutations in myelodysplastic syndrome are strongly correlated with aberrations of chromosome 5, and correlate with adverse prognosis. Br J Haematol 2013;160(5):660–72.

31. Takahashi K, Patel K, Bueso-Ramos C, et al. Clinical implications of TP53 mutations in myelodysplastic syndromes treated with hypomethylating agents. Oncotarget 2016;7(12):14172–87.

32. Sabapathy K, Lane DP. Therapeutic targeting of p53: all mutants are equal, but some mutants are more equal than others. Nat Rev Clin Oncol 2018;15(1): 13–30.

33. Kim MP, Zhang Y, Lozano G. Mutant p53: multiple mechanisms define biologic activity in cancer. Front Oncol 2015;5:249.

34. McGraw KL, Nguyen J, Komrokji RS, et al. Immunohistochemical pattern of p53 is a measure of TP53 mutation burden and adverse clinical outcome in myelodysplastic syndromes and secondary acute myeloid leukemia. Haematologica 2016;101(8):e320–3.

35. Haase D, Stevenson KE, Neuberg D, et al. TP53 mutation status divides myelodysplastic syndromes with complex karyotypes into distinct prognostic subgroups. Leukemia 2019;33(7):1747–58.

36. Walter MJ, Shen D, Shao J, et al. Clonal diversity of recurrently mutated genes in myelodysplastic syndromes. Leukemia 2013;27(6):1275–82.

37. Sallman DA, Komrokji R, Vaupel C, et al. Impact of TP53 mutation variant allele frequency on phenotype and outcomes in myelodysplastic syndromes. Leukemia 2016;30(3):666–73.

38. Sebaa A, Ades L, Baran-Marzack F, et al. Incidence of 17p deletions and TP53 mutation in myelodysplastic syndrome and acute myeloid leukemia with 5q deletion. Genes Chromosomes Cancer 2012;51(12):1086–92.

39. Jadersten M, Saft L, Smith A, et al. TP53 mutations in low-risk myelodysplastic syndromes with del(5q) predict disease progression. J Clin Oncol 2011;29(15): 1971–9.

40. Meggendorfer M, Haferlach C, Kern W, et al. Molecular analysis of myelodysplastic syndrome with isolated deletion of the long arm of chromosome 5 reveals a specific spectrum of molecular mutations with prognostic impact: a study on 123 patients and 27 genes. Haematologica 2017;102(9):1502–10.

41. Hunter AM, Komrokji RS, Al Ali N, et al. Baseline and sequential molecular profiling predicts outcomes in patients with MDS and oligoblastic AML treated with hypomethylating agents. Paper presented at: 15th International Symposium on Myelodysplastic Syndromes. Copenhagen, May 8, 2019.

42. DiNardo CD, Pratz K, Pullarkat V, et al. Venetoclax combined with decitabine or azacitidine in treatment-naive, elderly patients with acute myeloid leukemia. Blood 2019;133(1):7–17.

43. Christiansen DH, Andersen MK, Pedersen-Bjergaard J. Mutations with loss of heterozygosity of p53 are common in therapy-related myelodysplasia and acute myeloid leukemia after exposure to alkylating agents and significantly associated with deletion or loss of 5q, a complex karyotype, and a poor prognosis. J Clin Oncol 2001;19(5):1405–13.

44. Ok CY, Patel KP, Garcia-Manero G, et al. TP53 mutation characteristics in therapy-related myelodysplastic syndromes and acute myeloid leukemia is similar to de novo diseases. J Hematol Oncol 2015;8:45.

45. Pedersen-Bjergaard J, Andersen MK, Andersen MT, et al. Genetics of therapy-related myelodysplasia and acute myeloid leukemia. Leukemia 2008;22(2):240–8.

46. Hollenbach PW, Nguyen AN, Brady H, et al. A comparison of azacitidine and decitabine activities in acute myeloid leukemia cell lines. PLoS One 2010;5(2):e9001.

47. Christman JK. 5-Azacytidine and 5-aza-2'-deoxycytidine as inhibitors of DNA methylation: mechanistic studies and their implications for cancer therapy. Oncogene 2002;21(35):5483–95.

48. Fenaux P, Mufti GJ, Hellstrom-Lindberg E, et al. Efficacy of azacitidine compared with that of conventional care regimens in the treatment of higher-risk myelodysplastic syndromes: a randomised, open-label, phase III study. Lancet Oncol 2009;10(3):223–32.

49. Kantarjian H, Issa JP, Rosenfeld CS, et al. Decitabine improves patient outcomes in myelodysplastic syndromes: results of a phase III randomized study. Cancer 2006;106(8):1794–803.

50. Lubbert M, Suciu S, Baila L, et al. Low-dose decitabine versus best supportive care in elderly patients with intermediate- or high-risk myelodysplastic syndrome (MDS) ineligible for intensive chemotherapy: final results of the randomized phase III study of the European Organisation for Research and Treatment of Cancer Leukemia Group and the German MDS Study Group. J Clin Oncol 2011;29(15):1987–96.

51. Steensma DP, Baer MR, Slack JL, et al. Multicenter study of decitabine administered daily for 5 days every 4 weeks to adults with myelodysplastic syndromes: the alternative dosing for outpatient treatment (ADOPT) trial. J Clin Oncol 2009;27(23):3842–8.

52. Yi L, Sun Y, Levine A. Selected drugs that inhibit DNA methylation can preferentially kill p53 deficient cells. Oncotarget 2014;5(19):8924–36.

53. Nieto M, Samper E, Fraga MF, et al. The absence of p53 is critical for the induction of apoptosis by 5-aza-2'-deoxycytidine. Oncogene 2004;23(3):735–43.

54. Welch JS, Petti AA, Miller CA, et al. TP53 and decitabine in acute myeloid leukemia and myelodysplastic syndromes. N Engl J Med 2016;375(21):2023–36.

55. Chang CK, Zhao YS, Xu F, et al. TP53 mutations predict decitabine-induced complete responses in patients with myelodysplastic syndromes. Br J Haematol 2017;176(4):600–8.

56. Falconi G, Fabiani E, Piciocchi A, et al. Somatic mutations as markers of outcome after azacitidine and allogeneic stem cell transplantation in higher-risk myelodysplastic syndromes. Leukemia 2019;33(3):785–90.

57. David A, Sallman NHAA,Yun S, et al. Clonal suppression of TP53 mutant MDS and oligoblastic AML with hypomethylating agent therapy improves overall survival. Paper presented at: 2018 American Society of Hematology Annual Meeting. San Diego, December 1, 2018.

58. Short NJ, Kantarjian HM, Loghavi S, et al. Treatment with a 5-day versus a 10-day schedule of decitabine in older patients with newly diagnosed acute myeloid leukaemia: a randomised phase 2 trial. Lancet Haematol 2019;6(1):e29–37.

59. Arber DA, Orazi A, Hasserjian R, et al. The 2016 revision to the World Health Organization classification of myeloid neoplasms and acute leukemia. Blood 2016; 127(20):2391–405.

60. List A, Dewald G, Bennett J, et al. Lenalidomide in the myelodysplastic syndrome with chromosome 5q deletion. N Engl J Med 2006;355(14):1456–65.

61. Stahl M, Zeidan AM. Lenalidomide use in myelodysplastic syndromes: insights into the biologic mechanisms and clinical applications. Cancer 2017;123(10): 1703–13.

62. Wei S, Chen X, McGraw K, et al. Lenalidomide promotes p53 degradation by inhibiting MDM2 auto-ubiquitination in myelodysplastic syndrome with chromosome 5q deletion. Oncogene 2013;32(9):1110–20.

63. Caceres G, McGraw K, Yip BH, et al. TP53 suppression promotes erythropoiesis in del(5q) MDS, suggesting a targeted therapeutic strategy in lenalidomide-resistant patients. Proc Natl Acad Sci U S A 2013;110(40):16127–32.

64. Martinez-Høyer S, Docking R, Chan S, et al. Mechanisms of resistance to lenalidomide in Del(5q) myelodysplastic syndrome patients. Blood 2015;126(23): 5228.

65. Schneider RK, Adema V, Heckl D, et al. Role of casein kinase 1A1 in the biology and targeted therapy of del(5q) MDS. Cancer Cell 2014;26(4):509–20.

66. Mossner M, Jann JC, Nowak D, et al. Prevalence, clonal dynamics and clinical impact of TP53 mutations in patients with myelodysplastic syndrome with isolated deletion (5q) treated with lenalidomide: results from a prospective multicenter study of the German MDS study group (GMDS). Leukemia 2016;30(9): 1956–9.

67. Lode L, Menard A, Flet L, et al. Emergence and evolution of TP53 mutations are key features of disease progression in myelodysplastic patients with lower-risk del(5q) treated with lenalidomide. Haematologica 2018;103(4):e143–6.

68. Mallo M, Del Rey M, Ibanez M, et al. Response to lenalidomide in myelodysplastic syndromes with del(5q): influence of cytogenetics and mutations. Br J Haematol 2013;162(1):74–86.

69. Rasmussen B, Nilsson L, Jädersten M, et al. A randomized phase II study of standard dose azacitidine alone or in combination with lenalidomide in high-risk MDS with a karyotype including Del(5q). Paper presented at: 23rd Congress of the European Hematology Associate. Stockholm, June 17, 2018.

70. Koreth J, Pidala J, Perez WS, et al. Role of reduced-intensity conditioning allogeneic hematopoietic stem-cell transplantation in older patients with de novo myelodysplastic syndromes: an international collaborative decision analysis. J Clin Oncol 2013;31(21):2662–70.

71. de Witte T, Hermans J, Vossen J, et al. Haematopoietic stem cell transplantation for patients with myelo-dysplastic syndromes and secondary acute myeloid leukaemias: a report on behalf of the Chronic Leukaemia Working Party of the European Group for Blood and Marrow Transplantation (EBMT). Br J Haematol 2000;110(3):620–30.

72. Saber W, Cutler CS, Nakamura R, et al. Impact of donor source on hematopoietic cell transplantation outcomes for patients with myelodysplastic syndromes (MDS). Blood 2013;122(11):1974–82.

73. Kindwall-Keller T, Isola LM. The evolution of hematopoietic SCT in myelodysplastic syndrome. Bone Marrow Transplant 2009;43(8):597–609.

74. Scott BL, Sandmaier BM, Storer B, et al. Myeloablative vs nonmyeloablative allogeneic transplantation for patients with myelodysplastic syndrome or acute

myelogenous leukemia with multilineage dysplasia: a retrospective analysis. Leukemia 2006;20(1):128–35.

75. Della Porta MG, Galli A, Bacigalupo A, et al. Clinical effects of driver somatic mutations on the outcomes of patients with myelodysplastic syndromes treated with allogeneic hematopoietic stem-cell transplantation. J Clin Oncol 2016; 34(30):3627–37.

76. Yoshizato T, Nannya Y, Atsuta Y, et al. Genetic abnormalities in myelodysplasia and secondary acute myeloid leukemia: impact on outcome of stem cell transplantation. Blood 2017;129(17):2347–58.

77. Cutler C. Transplantation for therapy-related, TP53-mutated myelodysplastic syndrome: not because we can, but because we should. Haematologica 2017;102(12):1970–1.

78. Duncavage EJ, Jacoby MA, Chang GS, et al. Mutation clearance after transplantation for myelodysplastic syndrome. N Engl J Med 2018;379(11):1028–41.

79. de Lima M, Giralt S, Thall PF, et al. Maintenance therapy with low-dose azacitidine after allogeneic hematopoietic stem cell transplantation for recurrent acute myelogenous leukemia or myelodysplastic syndrome: a dose and schedule finding study. Cancer 2010;116(23):5420–31.

80. Pusic I, Choi J, Fiala MA, et al. Maintenance therapy with decitabine after allogeneic stem cell transplantation for acute myelogenous leukemia and myelodysplastic syndrome. Biol Blood Marrow Transplant 2015;21(10):1761–9.

81. Craddock C, Jilani N, Siddique S, et al. Tolerability and clinical activity of posttransplantation azacitidine in patients allografted for acute myeloid leukemia treated on the RICAZA trial. Biol Blood Marrow Transplant 2016;22(2):385–90.

82. Oran B, Lima M, Garcia-Manero G, et al. Maintenance with 5-azacytidine for acute myeloid leukemia and myelodysplastic syndrome patients. Paper presented at: 2018 American Society of Hematology Annual Meeting. San Diego, December 3, 2018.

83. Li D, Marchenko ND, Moll UM. SAHA shows preferential cytotoxicity in mutant p53 cancer cells by destabilizing mutant p53 through inhibition of the HDAC6-Hsp90 chaperone axis. Cell Death Differ 2011;18(12):1904–13.

84. Bug G, Burchert A, Wagner EM, et al. Phase I/II study of the deacetylase inhibitor panobinostat after allogeneic stem cell transplantation in patients with high-risk MDS or AML (PANOBEST trial). Leukemia 2017;31(11):2523–5.

85. Origanti S, Cai SR, Munir AZ, et al. Synthetic lethality of Chk1 inhibition combined with p53 and/or p21 loss during a DNA damage response in normal and tumor cells. Oncogene 2013;32(5):577–88.

86. Ma CX, Cai S, Li S, et al. Targeting Chk1 in p53-deficient triple-negative breast cancer is therapeutically beneficial in human-in-mouse tumor models. J Clin Invest 2012;122(4):1541–52.

87. Gyorffy B, Bottai G, Lehmann-Che J, et al. TP53 mutation-correlated genes predict the risk of tumor relapse and identify MPS1 as a potential therapeutic kinase in TP53-mutated breast cancers. Mol Oncol 2014;8(3):508–19.

88. Lord CJ, Ashworth A. PARP inhibitors: synthetic lethality in the clinic. Science 2017;355(6330):1152–8.

89. Tomita Y, Marchenko N, Erster S, et al. WT p53, but not tumor-derived mutants, bind to Bcl2 via the DNA binding domain and induce mitochondrial permeabilization. J Biol Chem 2006;281(13):8600–6.

90. Deng X, Gao F, Flagg T, et al. Bcl2's flexible loop domain regulates p53 binding and survival. Mol Cell Biol 2006;26(12):4421–34.

91. Vo TT, Ryan J, Carrasco R, et al. Relative mitochondrial priming of myeloblasts and normal HSCs determines chemotherapeutic success in AML. Cell 2012; 151(2):344–55.

92. Pan R, Hogdal LJ, Benito JM, et al. Selective BCL-2 inhibition by ABT-199 causes on-target cell death in acute myeloid leukemia. Cancer Discov 2014; 4(3):362–75.

93. Konopleva M, Contractor R, Tsao T, et al. Mechanisms of apoptosis sensitivity and resistance to the BH3 mimetic ABT-737 in acute myeloid leukemia. Cancer Cell 2006;10(5):375–88.

94. Nechiporuk T, Kurtz SE, Nikolova O, et al. The TP53 apoptotic network is a primary mediator of resistance to BCL2 inhibition in AML cells. Cancer Discov 2019;9(7):910–25.

95. Guihard S, Ramolu L, Macabre C, et al. The NEDD8 conjugation pathway regulates p53 transcriptional activity and head and neck cancer cell sensitivity to ionizing radiation. Int J Oncol 2012;41(4):1531–40.

96. Xirodimas DP, Saville MK, Bourdon JC, et al. Mdm2-mediated NEDD8 conjugation of p53 inhibits its transcriptional activity. Cell 2004;118(1):83–97.

97. Malhab LJ, Descamps S, Delaval B, et al. The use of the NEDD8 inhibitor MLN4924 (Pevonedistat) in a cyclotherapy approach to protect wild-type p53 cells from MLN4924 induced toxicity. Sci Rep 2016;6:37775.

98. Lin JJ, Milhollen MA, Smith PG, et al. NEDD8-targeting drug MLN4924 elicits DNA rereplication by stabilizing Cdt1 in S phase, triggering checkpoint activation, apoptosis, and senescence in cancer cells. Cancer Res 2010;70(24): 10310–20.

99. Smith PG, Traore T, Grossman S, et al. Azacitidine/decitabine synergism with the NEDD8-activating enzyme inhibitor MLN4924 in pre-clinical AML models. Blood 2011;118(21):578.

100. Swords RT, Coutre S, Maris MB, et al. Pevonedistat, a first-in-class NEDD8-activating enzyme inhibitor, combined with azacitidine in patients with AML. Blood 2018;131(13):1415–24.

101. Alexandrova EM, Yallowitz AR, Li D, et al. Improving survival by exploiting tumour dependence on stabilized mutant p53 for treatment. Nature 2015; 523(7560):352–6.

102. Li D, Marchenko ND, Schulz R, et al. Functional inactivation of endogenous MDM2 and CHIP by HSP90 causes aberrant stabilization of mutant p53 in human cancer cells. Mol Cancer Res 2011;9(5):577–88.

103. Dennis M, Hills RK, Thomas I, et al. A randomised assessment of Ganetespib combined with low dose Ara-C versus low dose Ara-C in older patients with acute myeloid leukaemia: results of the LI-1 trial. Blood 2016;128(22):2827.

104. Nishioka C, Ikezoe T, Yang J, et al. Simultaneous inhibition of DNA methyltransferase and histone deacetylase induces p53-independent apoptosis via downregulation of Mcl-1 in acute myelogenous leukemia cells. Leuk Res 2011;35(7): 932–9.

105. Craddock CF, Houlton AE, Quek LS, et al. Outcome of azacitidine therapy in acute myeloid leukemia is not improved by concurrent vorinostat therapy but is predicted by a diagnostic molecular signature. Clin Cancer Res 2017; 23(21):6430–40.

106. Prebet T, Sun Z, Ketterling RP, et al. Azacitidine with or without Entinostat for the treatment of therapy-related myeloid neoplasm: further results of the E1905 North American Leukemia Intergroup study. Br J Haematol 2016;172(3):384–91.

107. Issa JP, Garcia-Manero G, Huang X, et al. Results of phase 2 randomized study of low-dose decitabine with or without valproic acid in patients with myelodysplastic syndrome and acute myelogenous leukemia. Cancer 2015;121(4): 556–61.

108. Kirschbaum M, Gojo I, Goldberg SL, et al. A phase 1 clinical trial of vorinostat in combination with decitabine in patients with acute myeloid leukaemia or myelodysplastic syndrome. Br J Haematol 2014;167(2):185–93.

109. Min C, Moore N, Shearstone JR, et al. Selective inhibitors of histone deacetylases 1 and 2 synergize with azacitidine in acute myeloid leukemia. PLoS One 2017;12(1):e0169128.

110. Ungerstedt JS. Epigenetic modifiers in myeloid malignancies: the role of histone deacetylase inhibitors. Int J Mol Sci 2018;19(10) [pii:E3091].

111. Moon SH, Huang CH, Houlihan SL, et al. p53 represses the mevalonate pathway to mediate tumor suppression. Cell 2019;176(3):564–80.e19.

112. Parrales A, Ranjan A, Iyer SV, et al. DNAJA1 controls the fate of misfolded mutant p53 through the mevalonate pathway. Nat Cell Biol 2016;18(11): 1233–43.

113. Martirosyan A, Clendening JW, Goard CA, et al. Lovastatin induces apoptosis of ovarian cancer cells and synergizes with doxorubicin: potential therapeutic relevance. BMC Cancer 2010;10:103.

114. Burke LP, Kukoly CA. Statins induce lethal effects in acute myeloblastic leukemia [corrected] cells within 72 hours. Leuk Lymphoma 2008;49(2):322–30.

115. Lambert JM, Gorzov P, Veprintsev DB, et al. PRIMA-1 reactivates mutant p53 by covalent binding to the core domain. Cancer Cell 2009;15(5):376–88.

116. Perdrix A, Najem A, Saussez S, et al. PRIMA-1 and PRIMA-1(Met) (APR-246): from mutant/wild type p53 reactivation to unexpected mechanisms underlying their potent anti-tumor effect in combinatorial therapies. Cancers (Basel) 2017;9(12) [pii:E172].

117. Nahi H, Merup M, Lehmann S, et al. PRIMA-1 induces apoptosis in acute myeloid leukaemia cells with p53 gene deletion. Br J Haematol 2006;132(2): 230–6.

118. Ali D, Jonsson-Videsater K, Deneberg S, et al. APR-246 exhibits anti-leukemic activity and synergism with conventional chemotherapeutic drugs in acute myeloid leukemia cells. Eur J Haematol 2011;86(3):206–15.

119. Deneberg S, Cherif H, Lazarevic V, et al. An open-label phase I dose-finding study of APR-246 in hematological malignancies. Blood Cancer J 2016;6(7): e447.

120. Lehmann S, Bykov VJ, Ali D, et al. Targeting p53 in vivo: a first-in-human study with p53-targeting compound APR-246 in refractory hematologic malignancies and prostate cancer. J Clin Oncol 2012;30(29):3633–9.

121. Sallman DA, DeZern AE, Steensma DP, et al. Phase 1b/2 combination study of APR-246 and azacitidine (AZA) in patients with TP53 mutant myelodysplastic syndromes (MDS) and acute myeloid leukemia (AML). Blood 2018;132(Suppl 1):3091.

122. Williams P, Basu S, Garcia-Manero G, et al. The distribution of T-cell subsets and the expression of immune checkpoint receptors and ligands in patients with newly diagnosed and relapsed acute myeloid leukemia. Cancer 2019;125(9): 1470–81.

123. Yang H, Bueso-Ramos C, DiNardo C, et al. Expression of PD-L1, PD-L2, PD-1 and CTLA4 in myelodysplastic syndromes is enhanced by treatment with hypomethylating agents. Leukemia 2014;28(6):1280–8.

124. Zajac M, Zaleska J, Dolnik A, et al. Analysis of the PD-1/PD-L1 axis points to association of unfavorable recurrent mutations with PD-L1 expression in AML. Blood 2016;128(22):1685.

125. Sallman DA, Amy M, Komrokji RS, et al. Immune checkpoint profiling of TP53 mutant and wild-type myeloid malignancies: TP53 mutations direct immune tolerance via an immunosuppressive phenotype. Blood 2017;130(Suppl 1):423.

126. Orskov AD, Treppendahl MB, Skovbo A, et al. Hypomethylation and upregulation of PD-1 in T cells by azacytidine in MDS/AML patients: a rationale for combined targeting of PD-1 and DNA methylation. Oncotarget 2015;6(11): 9612–26.

127. Davids MS, Kim HT, Bachireddy P, et al. Ipilimumab for patients with relapse after allogeneic transplantation. N Engl J Med 2016;375(2):143–53.

128. Daver N, Garcia-Manero G, Basu S, et al. Efficacy, safety, and biomarkers of response to azacitidine and nivolumab in relapsed/refractory acute myeloid leukemia: a nonrandomized, open-label, phase II study. Cancer Discov 2019;9(3): 370–83.

129. Guillermo Garcia-Manero M, Koji Sasaki MD, Guillermo Montalban-Bravo MD, et al. A phase II study of nivolumab or ipilimumab with or without azacitidine for patients with myelodysplastic syndrome (MDS). Paper presented at: 2018 American Society of Hematology Annual Meeting. San Diego, December 1, 2018.

130. Guillermo Garcia-Manero M, Guillermo Montalban-Bravo MD, Koji Sasaki MD, et al. Double immune checkpoint inhibitor blockade with nivolumab and ipilimumab with or without azacitidine in patients with myelodysplastic syndrome (MDS). Paper presented at: 2018 American Society of Hematology Annual Meeting. San Diego, December 1, 2018.

131. Chao MP, Weissman IL, Majeti R. The CD47-SIRPalpha pathway in cancer immune evasion and potential therapeutic implications. Curr Opin Immunol 2012;24(2):225–32.

132. Jaiswal S, Jamieson CH, Pang WW, et al. CD47 is upregulated on circulating hematopoietic stem cells and leukemia cells to avoid phagocytosis. Cell 2009; 138(2):271–85.

133. Majeti R, Chao MP, Alizadeh AA, et al. CD47 is an adverse prognostic factor and therapeutic antibody target on human acute myeloid leukemia stem cells. Cell 2009;138(2):286–99.

134. Feng D, Gip P, McKenna KM, et al. Combination treatment with 5F9 and azacitidine enhances phagocytic elimination of acute myeloid leukemia. Blood 2018; 132(Suppl 1):2729.

135. Sallman DA, Donnellan WB, Asch AS, et al. The first-in-class anti-CD47 antibody Hu5F9-G4 is active and well tolerated alone or with azacitidine in AML and MDS patients: initial phase 1b results. J Clin Oncol 2019;37(15_suppl):7009.

136. Hoseini SS, Cheung NK. Acute myeloid leukemia targets for bispecific antibodies. Blood Cancer J 2017;7(2):e522.

137. Hofmann S, Schubert ML, Wang L, et al. Chimeric antigen receptor (CAR) T cell therapy in acute myeloid leukemia (AML). J Clin Med 2019;8(2) [pii:E200].

138. Uy GL, Rettig MP, Vey N, et al. Phase 1 cohort expansion of flotetuzumab, a CD123×CD3 bispecific dart® protein in patients with relapsed/refractory acute myeloid leukemia (AML). Blood 2018;132(Suppl 1):764.

139. Uy GL, Godwin J, Rettig MP, et al. Preliminary results of a phase 1 study of flotetuzumab, a CD123 x CD3 bispecific dart® protein, in patients with relapsed/

refractory acute myeloid leukemia and myelodysplastic syndrome. Blood 2017; 130(Suppl 1):637.

140. Ravandi F, Stein AS, Kantarjian HM, et al. A phase 1 first-in-human study of AMG 330, an anti-CD33 bispecific T-cell engager (BiTE®) antibody construct, in relapsed/refractory acute myeloid leukemia (R/R AML). Blood 2018;132(Suppl 1):25.

141. Sallman DA, Brayer J, Sagatys EM, et al. NKG2D-based chimeric antigen receptor therapy induced remission in a relapsed/refractory acute myeloid leukemia patient. Haematologica 2018;103(9):e424–6.

142. Baumeister SH, Murad J, Werner L, et al. Phase I trial of autologous CAR T cells targeting NKG2D ligands in patients with AML/MDS and multiple myeloma. Cancer Immunol Res 2019;7(1):100–12.

143. Sallman DA, Kerre T, Poire X, et al. Remissions in relapse/refractory acute myeloid leukemia patients following treatment with NKG2D CAR-T therapy without a prior preconditioning chemotherapy. Blood 2018;132(Suppl 1):902.

144. Budde L, Song JY, Kim Y, et al. Remissions of acute myeloid leukemia and blastic plasmacytoid dendritic cell neoplasm following treatment with CD123-specific CAR T cells: a first-in-human clinical trial. Blood 2017;130(Suppl 1):811.

145. Wang QS, Wang Y, Lv HY, et al. Treatment of CD33-directed chimeric antigen receptor-modified T cells in one patient with relapsed and refractory acute myeloid leukemia. Mol Ther 2015;23(1):184–91.

146. Liu F, Cao Y, Pinz K, et al. First-in-human CLL1-CD33 compound CAR T cell therapy induces complete remission in patients with refractory acute myeloid leukemia: update on phase 1 clinical trial. Blood 2018;132(Suppl 1):901.

147. Cummins KD, Frey N, Nelson AM, et al. Treating relapsed/refractory (RR) AML with biodegradable anti-CD123 CAR modified T cells. Blood 2017;130(Suppl 1):1359.

Prospects for Venetoclax in Myelodysplastic Syndromes

Jacqueline S. Garcia, MD

KEYWORDS

• Venetoclax • MDS • Apoptosis • BCL-2

KEY POINTS

• Despite significant progress in the genetic heterogeneity of myelodysplastic syndrome (MDS), novel and effective therapies have lagged behind that of many other malignancies, including acute myeloid leukemia.

• Inhibition of BCL-2 has preclinical rationale in MDS.

• Targeting the apoptotic machinery is a promising therapeutic approach that is undergoing clinical investigation in myeloid malignancies.

• More work is needed to identify predictive biomarkers in MDS.

INTRODUCTION

Myelodysplastic syndromes (MDS) are a heterogeneous group of clonal hematopoietic stem cell disorder with a limited therapeutic arsenal and overall poor outcome without an allogeneic hematopoietic stem cell transplantation. Standard therapies include the hypomethylating agents (HMAs) azacitidine and decitabine, and, once therapy fails, further treatment options are limited, with low overall survival of less than 6 months. Despite progress on uncovering the genetic landscape of MDS, which has provided insights into disease pathophysiology and evolution into leukemia,[1,2] clinical advances in identifying effective therapeutic targets within these heterogeneous diseases has remained slow, particularly for patients with high-risk disease. Since 2006, there has not been a Food and Drug Administration approval for an MDS therapy, although luspatercept[3] may be well on its way toward approval for the treatment of adult patients with very-low-risk to intermediate-risk MDS–associated anemia who have ring sideroblasts and required red blood cell transfusions. Although there are promising inhibitors of splicing factors[4,5] and refolding agents for mutant TP53[6] that are still under investigation, small molecule inhibitors of the isocitrate dehydrogenase 1[7] and isocitrate dehydrogenase 2[8] have made further clinical progress but have not yet garnered approvals for the treatment of MDS. Alternative pathways that drive chemoresistance, including deregulation of apoptosis,

Dana-Farber Cancer Institute, Harvard Medical School, 450 Brookline Avenue, Dana 2054, Boston, MA 02215, USA
E-mail address: Jacqueline_garcia@dfci.harvard.edu

Hematol Oncol Clin N Am 34 (2020) 441–448
https://doi.org/10.1016/j.hoc.2019.10.005
0889-8588/20/© 2019 Elsevier Inc. All rights reserved.

represent fertile ground for clinical investigation, particularly on the heels of the recent success of venetoclax plus an HMA[9] or cytarabine[10] that resulted in accelerated approval for the treatment of patients diagnosed with acute myeloid leukemia (AML) who were unfit for intensive chemotherapy or aged 75 years or older. This article outlines recent scientific advances that are informing future efforts to use BCL-2 inhibitors in clonal myeloid malignancies.

BCL-2 FAMILY MEDIATES MITOCHONDRIAL APOPTOSIS

The intrinsic (mitochondria-mediated) apoptotic pathway is triggered in response to cellular damage and to most anticancer therapies. The BCL-2 family consists of both antiapoptotic proteins (BCL-2, BCL-xL, MCL-1, BCL-w, and BFL-1/A1) and proapoptotic effector proteins (BAX, BAK, and BOK), which share the conserved BH3 domain. The BCL-2 family members regulate the mitochondrial pathway of apoptosis by controlling mitochondrial outer membrane permeabilization (MOMP), considered to be the point of no return for apoptosis in most instances by the activation of caspases. MOMP is followed by the release of soluble proteins, such as cytochrome c. Antiapoptotic proteins sequester activators, such as BID and BIM, or effector proteins to prevent apoptosis.[11] Sensitizers, including BAD, HRK, PUMA, NOXA, BMF, and BIK, act as selective antagonists of antiapoptotic proteins and contain only the BH3 domain (referred as BH3 only proteins).[12] BCL-2 proteins can selectively bind to each other, which is critical to their function. Apoptosis of cancer cells can occur by inducing an up-regulation of proapoptotic proteins or be directly decreasing the antiapoptotic proteins to allow activator proteins to initiate MOMP. Venetoclax, a BH3 mimetic and oral selective BCL-2 inhibitor, binds to the BH3-binding groove of BCL-2 and displaces BIM and other BH3-only proteins that normally are sequestered by BCL-2.[13] BH3-only proteins are then free to activate proapoptotic effectors like BAX and BAK. On BAX/BAK activation, these proteins subsequently oligomerize at the mitochondria, triggering MOMP.

BIOLOGY OF BCL-2 IN MYELOID MALIGNANCIES

BCL-2 is commonly expressed in hematologic malignancies.[14] Gene expression and protein levels of the antiapoptotic BCL-2 family members provided initial insights into the apoptotic pathway vulnerabilities in myeloid malignancies. For instance, reduced BIM gene expression was detected in higher-risk MDS, highlighting a potential therapeutic opportunity with proapoptotic BH3 mimetic drugs, such as venetoclax (ABT-199, Abbvie, and GDC-0199).[15] The exact mechanism determining the dysregulation of apoptotic induction in MDS is not yet fully detailed. Differential expression of antiapoptotic BCL-2 family members at different stages of MDS contribute to disease progression and chemoresistance. Aberrant splicing of these BCL-2 family members contributes to disease progression.[16] The level of apoptosis in low-risk MDS is higher than that observed in high-risk MDS/secondary AML or in healthy bone marrow mononuclear cells.[17] The ratio of proapoptotic (BAX/BAD) compared with that of antiapoptotic proteins (BCL-2/BCL-xL) in low-risk and high-risk MDS cases showed that disease progression was associated with significantly reduced ratios, primarily resulting from increased BCL-2 expression.[17] This exemplifies that malignant MDS cells acquire apoptotic resistance on disease progression. BCL-2 and BCL-xL overexpression in quiescent CD34+ leukemic cells further suggests the role of defective regulators of apoptosis in chemoresistance and a mechanism of protection for leukemic cells from proapoptotic stimuli.[18,19] Compared with bone marrows from healthy controls and low-risk MDS patients, in vitro treatment with BH3 mimetic

ABT-737, which binds to BCL-2, BCL-xL, and BCL-w, and ABT-199 in MDS patients resulted in elimination of primary stem/progenitor cells and differentiated bone marrow cells from high-risk MDS/secondary AML patients.[15,20]

BH3 PROFILING REVEALS APOPTOTIC VULNERABILITIES IN CANCER CELLS

Gene and protein expression of BCL-2 family members inadequately captures sensitivity to BH3 mimetics. Functional characterization of BCL-2 family members reveals therapeutic vulnerabilities and the apoptotic roadblocks that must be overcome for success. A cell's threshold to undergoing mitochondrial apoptosis (indicating how primed a cell is) can be measured by BH3 profiling, which is a flow cytometry–based assay that exposes permeabilized cancer cells to synthetic BH3 peptides to measure cytochrome c release as an indicator of MOMP.[12,21] BH3 profiling reveals how apoptotically primed a cell is compared with other cells, which can help differentiate cases where cells are primed for apoptosis due to the presence of antiapoptotic proteins that prevents BAX and BAK activation (responds to both activators and sensitizer BH3 peptides) from cells that are unprimed (responds to activators but minimal to no response to sensitizers) or potentially resistant due to loss of BAX and BAK function (no response to activators even at high doses).[21,22] Differential priming exists between myeloblasts and normal hematopoietic stem cells.[23] Apoptotic priming measured by BH3 profiling of pretreatment myeloblasts correlates with cytotoxic induction chemotherapy success in AML.[23]

Dependence on antiapoptotic BCL-2 family proteins can be inferred based on cytochrome c response to select sensitizers; specifically, cytochrome c release in response to the BH3 peptides BAD, HRK, and NOXA indicates dependence on BCL-2 and BCL-xL, BCL-xL, and MCL-1, respectively. Disease heterogeneity likely has an impact on differential BCL-2 family expression. Despite the presence of adverse genetic mutations, such as ASXL1, RUNX1, TP53, and EZH2, ABT-199 still induced apoptosis in progenitor cells from high-risk MDS/secondary AML cases, although gene expression levels of BCL-2, MCL-1, and BCL-xL did not vary significantly, suggesting that factors that influence priming are likely independent from underlying somatic mutations.[24]

PRECLINICAL DATA WITH VENETOCLAX IN MYELOID MALIGNANCIES

Venetoclax blocks the activity of the antiapoptotic prosurvival BCL-2 protein, which reduces the apoptotic threshold among myeloblasts. AML cell lines, primary patient samples, and murine primary xenografts were very sensitive to ABT-199, with death seen in less than 2 hours, consistent with the ex vivo sensitivity observed in chronic lymphocytic leukemia.[13] BH3 profiling confirmed activity at the level of the mitochondrion that correlated with treatment response. Because HMA therapy is the only approved therapy for high-risk MDS, adding select therapies that increase the antileukemic activity of these drugs is of highest priority. RNA-interference drug modifier screens identified antiapoptotic BCL-2 family members as potential targets of azacitidine-sensitization.[25] Although increased synergy with azacitidine was observed with ABT-737 compared with ABT-199, ABT-737 is not orally bioavailable. Combination therapy of venetoclax and azacitidine is a promising approach in myeloid malignancies as demonstrated in AML,[9] but data from patients with HMA failure are limited. Regimens that induce bone marrow suppression are particularly concerning as they relate to MDS, given the increased risk of toxicity, such as infectious complications from febrile neutropenia. In vitro data evaluating the impact of the combining of venetoclax and azacitidine on the viability of bone marrow mononuclear cells from patients with MDS/AML demonstrate that this regimen spares healthy hematopoietic cells.[26] BCL-2 expression among discrete leukemia subsets likely protects leukemic cells from oxidative stress and differential expression of BCL-2 along with reactive oxygen species level impact treatment resistance.[27,28] In particular, analysis of leukemia stem cells from patients treated with azacitidine and venetoclax revealed disruption in the metabolic pathway, specifically in the tricarboxylic acid cycle where decreased α-ketoglutarate and increased succinate levels were observed.[29]

CLINICAL DATA WITH SINGLE-AGENT VENETOCLAX IN ACUTE MYELOID LEUKEMIA

In a phase II venetoclax monotherapy trial for relapsed/refractory AML, the complete remission (CR) plus CR with incomplete blood count recovery (CRi) rate was 19% (6 of 32 patients), with most responses occurring by the end of 1 month.[30] Of these 32 patients treated on study, 41% (13 of 32 patients) reported an antecedent hematologic disorder or myeloproliferative neoplasm (further delineation of how many had prior MDS was not available). A majority of treated patients (72%, 23 of 32 patients) had received at least 1 prior HMA. Notably, half of the responders (3 of 6 patients) had an antecedent hematologic disorder (unspecified) and 25% of those who received prior HMA achieved CR/CRi. Common adverse events (AEs) included nausea, diarrhea, vomiting, febrile neutropenia, and hypokalemia. Specifically, febrile neutropenia was observed in 28% (9 of 32 patients). Tumor lysis syndrome was not seen.

CLINICAL VENETOCLAX COMBINATION STUDIES REVEAL THERAPEUTIC POTENTIAL IN MYELODYSPLASTIC SYNDROMES

A phase Ib study examined venetoclax in combination with the HMA azacitidine for the treatment of newly diagnosed AML for patients ineligible for intensive chemotherapy and not previously exposed to HMA therapy.[9] Combination therapy resulted in a striking CR plus CRi rate of 73% in the venetoclax, 400 mg, plus HMA cohort, which led to its accelerated approval on November 21, 2018 by the US Food and Drug Administration, with continued approval contingent on confirmatory trials (NCT02993523).[9] Although the number of patients with prior or underlying MDS was similarly not explicitly reported, nearly a quarter of the study population (36 of 145 patients) had a prior hematologic disorder and the response did not differ among those with de novo and secondary AML. These practice-changing results raise the tantalizing question of whether this combination has activity in related diseases, such as MDS. Although no dose-limiting toxicities, including laboratory or clinical tumor lysis syndrome, were observed,[9] most gastrointestinal AEs were grade 1 or grade 2, and common grade 3 or grade 4 AEs included febrile neutropenia (43%), neutropenia (17%), thrombocytopenia (24%), and pneumonia (13%). Other infectious-related complications, including bacteremia and sepsis, were reported in 10% of patients whereas grade 3 or grade 4 fungal infections were reported in only 8% of patients. Seven percent of deaths resulted from infections, including single cases of bacteremia, lung infection, fungal pneumonia septic shock, necrotizing pneumonia, and Pseudomonas sepsis, and 2 cases of both pneumonia and sepsis. These AEs altogether are not surprising given the underlying disease and toxicities known to be associated with HMA use.[31] Venetoclax was allowed to be interrupted for up to 14 days to allow for count recovery and thus cycle 2 of treatment was commonly delayed. Recurrent neutropenia events resulted in a dose reduction of venetoclax to 21 days for subsequent cycles and/or azacitidine dose reduction per package insert. In a parallel phase Ib/II study of venetoclax plus low-dose cytarabine[10] for patients 60 years or older with previously untreated AML ineligible for intensive chemotherapy, patients with prior treatment of

MDS with HMA were allowed. Approximately half of the study population (49%; 40 of 82 patients) had secondary AML and 29% had prior HMA treatment. The combined CR plus CRi rate of low-dose cytarabine with venetoclax (dosed at 600 mg daily continuously) was 54% with median time to response of 1.4 months, with a median overall survival of 10.1 months. Expectedly, patients with prior HMA exposure had a lower response rate with therapy (CR + CRi rate of 33%). From limited subsequent real-world retrospective analysis for patients treated at the MD Anderson Cancer Center (Houston, TX), 1 of 2 MDS patients responded to HMA plus venetoclax who was particularly heavily pretreated with prior HMA therapy and 2 prior allogeneic transplantations characterized by the adverse risk TP53 and RUNX1 mutations.[32] In a retrospective analysis of patients treated at City of Hope (Duarte, CA), 11 MDS patients were treated with HMA plus venetoclax and a third of patients (7 of 22 patients) with secondary AML achieved a CR/CRi.[33]

VENETOCLAX-BASED MYELODYSPLASTIC SYNDROME CLINICAL TRIALS ARE UNDER WAY

Clinical safety and activity of venetoclax as a single agent or in combination with azacitidine are under clinical investigation in the upfront (NCT02942290) and HMA refractory (NCT02966782) treatment settings for patients with MDS, with report of initial results presented at the American Society of Hematology meeting by December 2019. A chief concern about adding venetoclax to azacitidine in the MDS setting is the potential for prolonged neutropenia and associated infectious complications, which were reported in the phase Ib study of frontline venetoclax in combination with azacitidine for AML.[9] To minimize the risk of febrile neutropenia complications, these MDS study protocols were amended to reduce the duration of venetoclax exposure (continuous 14 days vs 28 days) to allow for hematologic recovery. Furthermore, similar to the AML studies, dose modifications were implemented to reduce the dose of venetoclax and azacitidine in the event of recurrent prolonged neutropenia. In addition to these studies, the safety of adding venetoclax to conditioning chemotherapy in patients with high-risk features in MDS, MDS/MPN, or AML undergoing reduced-intensity conditioning (RIC) chemotherapy for allogeneic stem cell transplantation (NCT03613532) is under way. The success of RIC-based transplantation relies primarily on the delayed graft-versus-leukemia effect but often is stymied by the presence of measurable residual disease at the time of transplantation that can expand and lead to disease relapse in the post-transplant setting.[34,35] This study asks if the addition of venetoclax can safely increase the antileukemic activity of RIC chemotherapy without impeding granulocyte engraftment, with the goal of ultimately thwarting impending relapse in a high-risk population. The addition of therapies to RIC regimens is not unique however, venetoclax does not require P53 dependent signaling to directly initiate apoptosis, has previously been shown to increase anti-leukemic activity when partnered with other active agents, and it has a relatively benign toxicity profile suggesting this approach might be a therapeutic opportunity.

Exploratory biomarkers for response to be considered in future venetoclax-based investigations include genetic analysis, BH3 profiling, and phospho-flow cytometry to measure protein abundance of BCL-2 family members. Exploratory BH3 profiling in the venetoclax monotherapy study was particularly useful in identifying responders based on inverse correlation with BCL-xL and MCL-1 proteins.[30] The combination of the measurements of BCL-2, BCL-xL and MCL-1 (mean fluorescence intensity of BCL-2/[BCL-xL + MCL-1]) in the subset of CD34$^+$ stem/progenitor cells among patients with high-risk MDS/secondary AML strongly associated with sensitivity to venetoclax.[24] The dynamic BH3 profiling (DBP) assay is another promising biomarker that offers insight into specific drug-induced death signaling after short-term ex vivo drug treatment of tumor cells and provides a rapid read-out of the change in apoptotic priming.[36] Results from DBP correlate with in vivo response to chemotherapy both in humans and in mice.[36,37] DBP of MDS cells may be another opportunity for identifying novel therapies either as a single agent or in combination with venetoclax. It is likely the combination of genetic and functional novel biomarkers will help optimize the use of BH3 mimetics, such as venetoclax, by identifying patients who will benefit most.

SUMMARY

Strong preclinical data and clinical trials, including venetoclax-based regimens in AML, provides therapeutic opportunity for patients with high-risk MDS. This article outlines the role of BCL-2 in myeloid malignancies and the clinical data and rationale for combination with HMA in AML and discusses correlative studies that highlight the pharmacodynamics of treatment response. Although results from ongoing early-phase clinical trials of venetoclax in combination with HMA in MDS are eagerly awaited, the author's current approach to maximize survival is to offer clinical trials to patients with high-risk disease in the upfront setting when appropriate and to all patients with HMA refractory disease. Remaining questions include whether activity in the upfront treatment of high-risk MDS will be as robust as they are in AML and the identification of other targeted therapies and chemotherapies with venetoclax are likely to be active in MDS.

DISCLOSURE

J.S. Garcia has received research support from Abbvie, Genentech, and Pfizer and serves on the scientific advisory board for Abbvie.

REFERENCES

1. da Silva-Coelho P, Kroeze LI, Yoshida K, et al. Clonal evolution in myelodysplastic syndromes. Nat Commun 2017;8:15099.
2. Makishima H, Yoshizato T, Yoshida K, et al. Dynamics of clonal evolution in myelodysplastic syndromes. Nat Genet 2017;49(2):204–12.
3. Fenaux P, Kiladjian JJ, Platzbecker U. Luspatercept for the treatment of anemia in myelodysplastic syndromes and primary myelofibrosis. Blood 2019;133(8): 790–4.
4. Steensma DP, Klimek VM, Yang J, et al. Phase I dose escalation clinical trial of H3B-8800, a splicing modulator, in patients with advanced myeloid malignancies. European Hematology Association Annual Meeting. Amsterdam 2019.
5. Lee SC, Dvinge H, Kim E, et al. Modulation of splicing catalysis for therapeutic targeting of leukemia with mutations in genes encoding spliceosomal proteins. Nat Med 2016;22(6):672–8.
6. Sallman DA, deZern AE, Sweet K, et al. Phase 1B/2 combination study of APR-246 and azacitidine (AZA) in patients with TP53 mutant myelodysplastic syndromes (MDS) and acute myeloid leukemia (AML). 23rd Congress of the European Hematology Association. Stockholm 2018.
7. DiNardo CD, Stein EM, de Botton S, et al. Durable remissions with Ivosidenib in IDH1-mutated relapsed or refractory AML. N Engl J Med 2018;378(25):2386–98.
8. Stein EM, DiNardo CD, Pollyea DA, et al. Enasidenib in mutant IDH2 relapsed or refractory acute myeloid leukemia. Blood 2017;130(6):722–31.

9. DiNardo CD, Pratz K, Pullarkat V, et al. Venetoclax combined with decitabine or azacitidine in treatment-naive, elderly patients with acute myeloid leukemia. Blood 2019;133(1):7–17.

10. Wei AH, Strickland SA Jr, Hou JZ, et al. Venetoclax combined with low-dose cytarabine for previously untreated patients with acute myeloid leukemia: results from a Phase Ib/II study. J Clin Oncol 2019;37(15):1277–84.

11. Cheng EH, Wei MC, Weiler S, et al. BCL-2, BCL-X(L) sequester BH3 domain-only molecules preventing BAX- and BAK-mediated mitochondrial apoptosis. Mol Cell 2001;8(3):705–11.

12. Certo M, Del Gaizo Moore V, Nishino M, et al. Mitochondria primed by death signals determine cellular addiction to antiapoptotic BCL-2 family members. Cancer Cell 2006;9(5):351–65.

13. Pan R, Hogdal LJ, Benito JM, et al. Selective BCL-2 inhibition by ABT-199 causes on-target cell death in acute myeloid leukemia. Cancer Discov 2014;4(3):362–75.

14. Adams JM, Cory S. The Bcl-2 apoptotic switch in cancer development and therapy. Oncogene 2007;26(9):1324–37.

15. Jilg S, Reidel V, Muller-Thomas C, et al. Blockade of BCL-2 proteins efficiently induces apoptosis in progenitor cells of high-risk myelodysplastic syndromes patients. Leukemia 2016;30(1):112–23.

16. Crews LA, Balaian L, Delos Santos NP, et al. RNA splicing modulation selectively impairs leukemia stem cell maintenance in secondary human AML. Cell Stem Cell 2016;19(5):599–612.

17. Parker JE, Mufti GJ, Rasool F, et al. The role of apoptosis, proliferation, and the Bcl-2-related proteins in the myelodysplastic syndromes and acute myeloid leukemia secondary to MDS. Blood 2000;96(12):3932–8.

18. Konopleva M, Zhao S, Hu W, et al. The anti-apoptotic genes Bcl-X(L) and Bcl-2 are over-expressed and contribute to chemoresistance of non-proliferating leukaemic CD34+ cells. Br J Haematol 2002;118(2):521–34.

19. Tacke F, Marini FC 3rd, Zhao S, et al. Expression of inducible Bcl-X(S) in myeloid leukemia: compensatory upregulation of Bcl-X(L) and Bcl-2 prevents apoptosis and chemosensitization. Cancer Biol Ther 2004;3(3):340–7.

20. Oltersdorf T, Elmore SW, Shoemaker AR, et al. An inhibitor of Bcl-2 family proteins induces regression of solid tumours. Nature 2005;435(7042):677–81.

21. Deng J, Carlson N, Takeyama K, et al. BH3 profiling identifies three distinct classes of apoptotic blocks to predict response to ABT-737 and conventional chemotherapeutic agents. Cancer Cell 2007;12(2):171–85.

22. Letai A, Bassik MC, Walensky LD, et al. Distinct BH3 domains either sensitize or activate mitochondrial apoptosis, serving as prototype cancer therapeutics. Cancer Cell 2002;2(3):183–92.

23. Vo TT, Ryan J, Carrasco R, et al. Relative mitochondrial priming of myeloblasts and normal HSCs determines chemotherapeutic success in AML. Cell 2012;151(2):344–55.

24. Reidel V, Kauschinger J, Hauch RT, et al. Selective inhibition of BCL-2 is a promising target in patients with high-risk myelodysplastic syndromes and adverse mutational profile. Oncotarget 2018;9(25):17270–81.

25. Bogenberger JM, Kornblau SM, Pierceall WE, et al. BCL-2 family proteins as 5-Azacytidine-sensitizing targets and determinants of response in myeloid malignancies. Leukemia 2014;28(8):1657–65.

26. Jilg S, Hauch RT, Kauschinger J, et al. Venetoclax with azacitidine targets refractory MDS but spares healthy hematopoiesis at tailored dose. Exp Hematol Oncol 2019;8:9.

27. Khan N, Hills RK, Knapper S, et al. Normal hematopoietic progenitor subsets have distinct reactive oxygen species, BCL2 and cell-cycle profiles that are decoupled from maturation in acute myeloid leukemia. PLoS One 2016;11(9): e0163291.

28. Lagadinou ED, Sach A, Callahan K, et al. BCL-2 inhibition targets oxidative phosphorylation and selectively eradicates quiescent human leukemia stem cells. Cell Stem Cell 2013;12(3):329–41.

29. Pollyea DA, Stevens BM, Jones CL, et al. Venetoclax with azacitidine disrupts energy metabolism and targets leukemia stem cells in patients with acute myeloid leukemia. Nat Med 2018;24(12):1859–66.

30. Konopleva M, Pollyea DA, Potluri J, et al. Efficacy and biological correlates of response in a Phase II study of venetoclax monotherapy in patients with acute myelogenous leukemia. Cancer Discov 2016;6(10):1106–17.

31. Fenaux P, Mufti GJ, Hellstrom-Lindberg E, et al. Efficacy of azacitidine compared with that of conventional care regimens in the treatment of higher-risk myelodysplastic syndromes: a randomised, open-label, phase III study. Lancet Oncol 2009;10(3):223–32.

32. DiNardo CD, Rausch CR, Benton C, et al. Clinical experience with the BCL2-inhibitor venetoclax in combination therapy for relapsed and refractory acute myeloid leukemia and related myeloid malignancies. Am J Hematol 2018;93(3): 401–7.

33. Aldoss I, Yang D, Aribi A, et al. Efficacy of the combination of venetoclax and hypomethylating agents in relapsed/refractory acute myeloid leukemia. Haematologica 2018;103(9):e404–7.

34. Thol F, Gabdoulline R, Liebich A, et al. Measurable residual disease monitoring by NGS before allogeneic hematopoietic cell transplantation in AML. Blood 2018;132(16):1703–13.

35. Walter RB, Gooley TA, Wood BL, et al. Impact of pretransplantation minimal residual disease, as detected by multiparametric flow cytometry, on outcome of myeloablative hematopoietic cell transplantation for acute myeloid leukemia. J Clin Oncol 2011;29(9):1190–7.

36. Montero J, Sarosiek KA, DeAngelo JD, et al. Drug-induced death signaling strategy rapidly predicts cancer response to chemotherapy. Cell 2015;160(5):977–89.

37. Townsend EC, Murakami MA, Christodoulou A, et al. The public repository of xenografts enables discovery and randomized phase II-like trials in mice. Cancer Cell 2016;29(4):574–86.

Secondary Acute Myeloid Leukemia

A Primary Challenge of Diagnosis and Treatment

Eric S. Winer, MD

KEYWORDS

- Acute myeloid leukemia • Secondary acute myeloid leukemia
- Therapy-related acute myeloid leukemia
- Acute Myeloid Leukemia Caused by an Antecedent Hematologic Disease
- Acute Myeloid Leukemia with Myelodysplastic-Related Changes

KEY POINTS

- Secondary acute myeloid leukemia (sAML) is a unique diagnostic entity with specific clinical and laboratory characteristics.
- sAML independently carries a poor prognosis.
- Challenges to treating the sAML population include high rate of comorbidities in patients and chemorefractory disease.
- Improvement in molecular diagnostics and novel therapies will lead to improved outcomes in this high-risk population.

INTRODUCTION

Acute myeloid leukemia (AML) is a heterogenous, aggressive myeloid malignancy. In 2018, an estimated 19,520 new cases and 10,670 deaths occurred in the United States.[1] Although strides have been made in AML treatment using novel therapies and small molecule inhibitors, the 5-year overall survival (OS) is only approximately 27%.[2,3] Contributing to this dismal prognosis is the increasing rates of secondary AML (sAML), which describe a subset of AML that arises from either an antecedent hematologic disorder (AHD) such as myelodysplastic syndrome (MDS), or are related to prior exposure to cytotoxic chemotherapy agents or radiation therapy. The incidence of sAML ranges from 10% to 35% of AML cases.[4,5] This article focuses on the epidemiology, diagnosis, pathogenesis, molecular, and treatment of sAML.

Adult Leukemia Program, Department of Medical Oncology, Dana Farber Cancer Institute, 450 Brookline Avenue, Boston, MA 02215, USA
E-mail address: erics_winer@dfci.harvard.edu

Hematol Oncol Clin N Am 34 (2020) 449–463
https://doi.org/10.1016/j.hoc.2019.11.003
0889-8588/20/© 2019 Elsevier Inc. All rights reserved.

hemonc.theclinics.com

DIAGNOSIS AND CLASSIFICATION

Secondary AML occurs by 2 separate mechanisms, either through an antecedent he-matologic disorder (AHD) or prior chemotherapy or radiation therapy, and the classi-fication of AML has begun to reflect this etiology.[6] In a study evaluating the ontogeny of AML, distinct somatic mutations differentiated AML subtypes between de novo AML, AML-AHD (labeled as s-AML), and therapy-related AML (t-AML).[7] Multiple ana-lyses have been studied to determine the transformational cause for the change from AHD to AML. Clonal evolution in AML is common, with many of the mutations occur-ring as random events, then acquiring a cooperating mutation leading to proliferation of the malignant clone.[8] In 2008, the World Health Organization (WHO) introduced the diagnosis of AML with myelodysplasia-related changes (AML-MRC), which was later expanded to specific criteria in the 2016 WHO classification system.[6,9] This newer classification requires a prior history of MDS, MDS-associated cytogenetic abnormal-ities, or multilineage dysplasia, but specifically excludes prior cytotoxic chemotherapy or radiation therapy and entity-defining recurring cytogenetic abnormalities.[10] The classification of AML-MRC has a high frequency of mutations in ASXL1 mutations, and a low rating of NPM1, FLT3, and DNMT3A mutations.[11] Patients with AML-MRC who have either the ASXL1 mutation or TP53 mutations are associated with shorter OS.[12] In a retrospective study of Chinese patients with AML-MRC, patients had significantly shortened complete response (CR) rates, disease-free survival (DFS), and OS compared with AML-NOS patients.[13]

PATHOPHYSIOLOGY

t-AML is defined as AML occurring in patients previously treated with chemotherapy, radiation therapy, or immunosuppressive therapy.[14] The incidence of therapy-related MDS (t-MDS) and t-AML ranges from 0.8% to 6.3% at 20 years, with a marked decrease in incidence after 10 years.[15] The classic teachings associate t-AML with alkylating agents, with a latency period of 5 years, and topoisomerase II inhibitors, with a latency period of 1.5 years.[16,17] Radiation also is associated with t-AML, as demonstrated by an Italian breast cancer study that controlled for chemotherapy treatment regimens.[18] In a large case-controlled study in breast cancer, the risk of AML was far higher in patients receiving alkylating agents alone (relative risk [RR] 10.0) than with radiation alone (RR 2.4), but the combination displayed the highest risk (RR 17.4%).[19]

Unique chromosomal abnormalities frequently occur with t-AML. A large Swedish pooled analysis demonstrated an increase in complex and hypodiploid karyotypes. Furthermore, certain chromosomal abnormalities corresponded with specific treat-ments, such as 5q- and radiotherapy, monosomy 7 and monosomy 5 with alkylating agents, and t(11q23) and other balanced translocations with topoisomerase II inhibi-tors.[20,21] Not surprisingly, combination chemoradiation therapy has the highest inci-dence of t-AML, and a higher frequency of complex karyotype.[22] The prognosis of t-AML depends on these cytogenetic abnormalities.[23]

Molecular studies have also elucidated the pathway of t-AML. Point mutations in AML1 and RAS seem to predispose the patient to progression from t-MDS to AML.[21] However, the most commonly mutated gene in t-AML is TP53, occurring in 37% of t-MDS/t-AML cases compared with 14.5% of de novo MDS/AML cases.[24] It is well established that TP53 is associated with leukemogenesis and complex karyo-type, and is associated with poor prognosis.[25,26] One theory of p53 pathogenesis is that a small percentage of patients is predisposed to TP53 selection by possessing mutations as clonal hematopoiesis of indeterminate potential.[27] In a small study evaluating 22 patients with t-AML, 4 patients had the exact founder mutation at diagnosis that was also present at low frequencies (0.003%–0.7%) in mobilized peripheral leukocytes or bone marrow 3 to 6 years before the development of t-AML; in 2 cases, patients had the founder TP53 mutation prior to initiation of chemotherapy.[28] These data may indicate chemotherapy may not be a direct inducer of TP53 mutations, but rather a selector of the hematopoietic stem cells that possess the clonal age-related p53 mutation promoting expansion.

The remainder of sAML is associated with an AHD. This includes MDS, aplastic anemia, and the myeloproliferative diseases, including chronic myeloid leukemia, polycythemia vera, primary myelofibrosis, and essential thrombocythemia.[29] MDS is a heterogeneous diagnosis; in low-risk MDS with refractory anemia, approximately 2% of cases will transform to AML, while in the subset with excess blasts-2, approximately 40% will progress to AML at 5 years.[30] The transformation process from MDS to AML is slowly being elucidated. In 1 study, whole-genome sequencing demonstrated a clonal evolution with nearly all bone marrow cells in patients with MDS and sAML being clonally derived, with 1 of 11 distinct mutations acquired in addition to the antecedent founder clone.[31] Further studies evaluating the progression from MDS to sAML in paired samples demonstrated that 60% of patients acquired additional mutations (24% cytogenetic, 26% molecular, 11% both) leading to the progression from MDS to sAML.[32] Furthermore, although specific genes are common in the initiation of MDS, such as SRSF2, SF3B1, U2AF1, ZRSR2, ASXL1, EZH2, BCOR, and STAG2, the addition of progression mutations such as RUNX1, GATA2, and CEBPA are often needed to evade normal cellular differentiation.[7] Other mutations, such as FLT3 and Ras family mutations often become the driver mutation to sAML because of the effect of dysregulation of cellular proliferation.[33] Often these comutations are from different classes of biologic function and create a pattern of functional complementarity.[34]

Further mutational analyses have attempted to clarify the transformation from MDS to sAML. RUNX1 is a common mutation in MDS, but seems to have an increased incidence in sAML.[35] A transcription factor essential for normal hematopoiesis, RUNX1 is seen in high frequency of CMML and MDS cases; RUNX1 mutants in these diagnoses have reduced DNA binding. This low RUNX1 activity correlated with both a higher risk and shorter time to the development of sAML.[36] DNMT3A mutations, typically found in de novo AML with mutations in the arginine on position 882, are also noted in sAML and can be found in the antecedent disorder, but the mutation is more frequently seen in the methyltransferase domain.[37] TET2 mutations, common in de novo MDS, occur more frequently in sAML compared with AML-MRC and did not associate with mutations of NPM1, FLT3, Ras, or WT1. In a multivariate large database analysis, there was noted linearity in the transformation curves from MDS to AML over time when the group was divided by IPSS subsets; this led investigators to hypothesize that duration of MDS may not be of prognostic relevance, but rather the transformation is caused by a single epigenetic or genetic event.[38] This concept of a single event leading to leukemogenesis in sAML patients was reported by Milosevic and colleagues,[39] who identified 36 recurrent aberrations.

Other secondary causes of AML are uncommon. Myeloproliferative neoplasms (MPNs) have a lower rate of transformation to sAML, and patients with transformation from JAK2 MPN have higher incidence of DNA methylation mutations (most commonly *ETV6, NRAS, BCOR, SF3B1, CBL, GATA2, RAD21, KRAS, ABL1* and *PTPN11*) and complex karyotype. TP53 was noted in both MPN-driven and de novo AML; a study evaluating the functional analysis of leukemic transformation in MPN demonstrated frequent acquisition of TP53 mutations.[40,41] Nonmalignancy diagnoses associated with sAML include chemical exposure such as benzene (odds ratio [OR] 1.77), vinyl chloride (OR 2.81), and other environmental exposures but into pesticides or agricultural chemicals.[42] A study evaluating autoimmune therapy such as azathioprine demonstrated an increase in sMDS/sAML (OR 7.05).[43] Lastly, there is a study suggesting that number of apheresis days prior to autologous stem cell transplantation for lymphoma may be a predictor of the development of sMDS/sMDS, but this may not be a causal effect but rather a predictive one.[44]

EPIDEMIOLOGY AND PROGNOSIS

Multiple studies have tried to elucidate the true incidence and other prognostic factors for s-AML. In a Swedish registry study including 3363 adult patients with AML, 639 (18.7%) had AHD-AML, while 259 (7.7%) had t-AML (**Table 1**).[45] A second population study from Denmark evaluated 3055 unselected patients and noted a frequency of sAML of 19.8% and of t-AML 6.6%.[5] The German-Austrian AMLSG surveyed 2653 AML patients and noted 200 (7.0%) to have t-AML; secondary AML data were not provided.[46] A Czech Republic study evaluated 1516 patients, 328 of whom were diagnosed with s-AML (21.6%), but this study did not differentiate between s-AML and t-AML. Descriptively, the s-AML population was older, had a higher frequency of unfavorable cytogenetics, and were less likely to receive curative therapy.[47]

Age carries a mixed prognosis in s-AML. In the Swedish study, there was not a significant difference in median age between s-AML and de novo AML (73 years vs 71 years); however, there was a significant difference in incidence below age 40.[45] Also, although younger patients tended to do well in de novo AML, survival was poor in s-AML and similar to the elderly patients (158 months vs 7–14 months in patients < 55). In the Czech study, the median age of s-AML patients was 5 years older, with a higher proportion of patients over the age of 60.[47] In the Danish study, patients under 60 had an increased relative risk for death in s-AML and t-AML, whereas in older patients, s-AML and t-AML had no impact on survival.[5] One further transplant study in sAML and MDS revealed an increase in significant complications and late treatment-related mortality for patients aged 65 years and older versus patients younger than 45 years of age.[48]

Response to chemotherapy and OS was heavily impacted by s-AML versus de novo AML. In the Czech study, the complete remission was achieved in only 48.9% of patients who received curative therapy compared with 74.6% of de novo AML cases (P<.001). Differences in OS were also noted in the groups achieving CR, with the s-AML group having a median OS of 14.1 months compared with 37.4 months in de novo AML.[47] The Danish study created subsets of s-AML from MDS (MDS-sAML), s-AML from other AHD (non-MDS-AML), and t-AML. All 3 categories had a worsened odds ratio to achieve a CR (MDS-sAML 0.47, non-MDS-sAML 0.39, t-AML 0.51).[5] The data from the Swedish study mimicked the aforementioned studies, with CR rates of 72% in de novo AML, but only 54% of t-AML and 39% in AHD-AML. A multivariable Cox regression analysis showed both AHD-AML and t-AML to be independently associated with poor survival (HR 1.51 and 1.72, respectively).[45]

Other studies present a retrospective report of their s-AML patients. The Duke University group evaluated 96 patients with AML treated with induction chemotherapy, and demonstrated a CR rate of 73%; patients with t-AML had a higher response rate (82%) compared with s-AML (62%). However, long-term prognosis was still poor, with an event free survival (EFS) of 8 months and OS of 13.6 months.[49] A second report from MD Anderson detailed s-AML strictly defined as prior MDS, MPN, or aplastic anemia, with at least 1 treatment for that diagnosis. CR rates and

Table 1
Characteristics of secondary acute myeloid leukemia

Author	N	Age	% Secondary Acute Myeloid Leukemia	Complete Response Rate with Intensive Chemotherapy	Survival	Other Data
Hulegårdh et al,[45] 2015	3363	17–98	18.7% AHD-AML 7.7% t-AML	72% de novo 39% AHD-AML 54% t-AML	Independent risk factor for poor survival AHD-AML HR 1.51 t-AML HR 1.72	Worse prognosis in younger population (<55) De novo: 158 mo AHD-AML: 7 mo t-AML: 14 mo
Szotkowski et al,[47] 2010	1516	19–92	21.6% sAML	74.6% de novo 48.9% sAML	Median OS: De novo: 18.2 mo sAML: 8.2 mo	Age and cytogenetics as independent risk factors for OS
Østgård et al,[5] 2015	3055	15–87	19.8% sAML (AHD) 6.6% t-AML	75% de novo 59% MDS-sAML 61% t-AML 54% non-MDS-sAML	1 y/3 y OS: de novo: 65%/39% MDS-sAML: 56%/25% t-AML: 45%/24% Non-MDS-sAML: 31%/11%	Non-MDS-AML as inferior survival across all age and cytogenetic risk groups
Boddu et al,[51] 2017	931	60–75	100%	46% with IC 45% with Vyxeos 36% with HMA 43% with LDAC	Median OS: IC: 5.4 mo Vyxeos: 7.6 mo HMA: 6.7 mo LDAC: 7.1 mo	Lower-intensity regimens in this older population had improved OS
Rizzieri et al,[49] 2009	96	22–82	100%	58% with IC	1 y OS: 51%	Median DFS of 11 mo.
Bertoli et al,[52] 2019	218	60–75	100%	CR/CRi 69.4% IC CR/CRi 15% HMA	Median OS: 11 mo IC 11 mo HMA	3 y/5 y OS: 21% and 17% IC 15% and 2% HMA

Abbreviations: AHD, antecedent hematologic disease; HMA, hypomethylating agent; t-AML, therapy-related AML.

8-week mortality rates were 32% and 27%, respectively in patients younger than 60 years and 24% and 19% respectively in patients aged 60 years and older.[50] In a companion study, the same group evaluated s-AML in older patients stratified by intensive chemotherapy (IC), hypomethylating-based therapy (HMA), low-dose cytarabine-based regimens (LDAC), Vyxeos (CPX-351), and investigational agents. CR rates were higher in the IC, Vyxeos, and LDAC arms compared with HMA, but the lower-intensity regimens (HMA and LDAC) had superior OS compared with IC (6.9 months vs 5.4 months).[51] A French study presented their experience with s-AML cases receiving either IC or HMA. The IC group achieved a CR rate of 69% and OS of 11 months, while the HMA group achieved a CR rate of 15%, but an identical median OS of 11 months. However, different 3- and 5-year OS rates were noted, with the IC group demonstrating 21% and 17% ,respectively compared with 15% and 2% in the HMA group.[52]

The German Study Alliance Leukemia (SAL) evaluated patients in the AML96 trial with sAML. This study found absolute platelet count and NPM1 gene mutation status as prognostic factors.[53] These risk factors were added to known risk factors of age and karyotype. This created 3 score groups that stratified 2-year OS and EFS of 53% and 44%, respectively, in the low-risk group, 21% and 12%, respectively, in the intermediate risk group, and 7% and 3%, respectively, in the high-risk group.

TREATMENT

Unfortunately, there are few prospective clinical trials that solely evaluate sAML, as it is a small subset of AML; often these patients are excluded from individual trials. Further complicating treatment strategies is that these patients have often received prior treatment for an antecedent hematologic disorder, exposing patients to commonly used agents for AML treatment (ie, hypomethylating agents in MDS) or increasing comorbidities by chemotherapies used in treating previous solid tumors.[16] Although recent advances in novel therapies created more therapeutic opportunities, these options have not been proven in sAML patients; therefore, further studies are needed in this unmet population.

Standard Therapy

For almost 50 years, the standard of care for fit AML patient was 7 + 3 chemotherapy, combining 7 days of cytarabine with 3 days of anthracycline.[54] Subsequent large randomized studies have attempted to tailor the dosing to maximize efficacy, but overall the response for all AML patients ranges from 54% to 82%.[55–58] The subsets of secondary AML patients were not part of any planned analyses, but some data were included in individual studies. In a study in patients over the age of 60 comparing daunorubicin at 45 mg/m^2 with 90 mg/m^2, the sAML patients, particularly with prior MDS, had a lower likelihood of achieving a complete remission (OR 0.44).[57] The British AML17 trial, which compared double induction daunorubicin 90 mg/m^2 with 60 mg/m^2 therapy did not demonstrate any difference in outcome from treatments in the de novo, secondary, or MDS groups.[58] A Korean study also evaluating daunorubicin at 45 mg/m^2 with 90 mg/m^2 had a small subset of sAML (4.4%) and noted a trend toward lower CR rates (de novo 78.1% vs 58.8%, $P = .63$).[55]

Other Traditional Chemotherapies

CPX-351 (Vyxeos) is a liposomal-encapsulated cytarabine:daunorubicin mixture at a 5:1 M ration, which effectively translates to 1 unit of CPX-351 containing 1 mg of cytarabine and 0.44 mg of daunorubicin. This novel delivery system maintains the 5:1 ratio, and the drug's synergistic effects and maximizes drug delivery to leukemic cells.[59] After a phase I dose escalation trial demonstrated safety,[60] The phase II study included older AML patients and randomized them to CPX-351 versus 7 + 3. CPX-351 yielded a higher CR rate (66.7% vs 51.2%) with no difference in EFS and OS. However, a planned subset analysis of sAML patients demonstrated improved although not statistically significant response rates (57.6% vs31.6%, $P = 0/06$) and prolongation of OS (HR $= 0.46$, $P=.01$).[61]

These promising results led to a phase III trial specific to untreated sAML.[62] The eligibility criteria included patients aged 60 to 75 years with either newly diagnosed t-AML, AML with antecedent MDS or CMML, or de novo AML with MDS-related cytogenetic abnormalities based on the 2008 WHO criteria. Patients who had previously received HMA were eligible, and the primary end point was survival. Patients were randomized to receive either CPX-351 at $100u/m^2$ or standard induction with cytarabine $100 mg/m^2$ and daunorubicin $60 mg/m^2$.

The results of this sAML trial were practice changing. Three hundred nine patients were randomized, and full analysis demonstrated in improved OS with CPX-351 compared with standard induction (9.56 months vs 5.95 months). Kaplan-Meier estimates favored the CPX-351 group (1-year OS 41.5% vs 27.6% and 2-year OS 31.1% vs 12.3%). The CR + CR rate with incomplete count recovery (CRi) also was higher in the CPX-351 arm compared with an underperforming 7 + 3 (47.7% vs 33.3%, $P=.04$). Rates of adverse events were similar between the 2 groups. Multiple subgroup analyses were evaluated in the study, with the survival benefit of CPX-351 consistent across all age groups, but nonsignificant differences noted in patients with MDS with prior HMA exposure (CPX-351 5.65 vs 7 + 3 7.32 months), de novo AML with MDS karyotype (10.09 vs 7.36 months), unfavorable cytogenetics (6.6 vs 5.16 months) FLT3 mutation (10.25 vs 4.6 months), and all prior HMA exposure (5.65 vs 5.9 months). Further subset analysis evaluated survival following allogeneic transplant and demonstrated that of the 91 patients transplanted, there was a higher 100-day mortality in the 7 + 3 group (20.5% vs 9.6%) and a markedly better OS in the CPX-351 arm (HR 0.46, $P=.0046$). These data led to US Food and Drug Administration (FDA) approval of CPX-351 in patients over 18 years of age with t-AML or AML-MRC.

A smaller study evaluated the use of CPX-351 at low doses 32 or 64 U/m^2 versus the standard 101 U/m^2 in a phase II study.[63] The sAML patients accounted for 55.3% of all patients. The 64 U/m^2 arm was stopped early because of 4 early deaths in the first 10 patients, and the remaining patients were treated at the 32 U/m^2 dose. Unfortunately, the ORR was only 26.3%, with a median OS of 3 months; the death rate within 28 days was 28.9%.

Other studies have attempted to determine a better conventional chemotherapy treatment for sAML. One study examined continuous fludarabine with cytarabine and G-CSF (FLAG) in elderly patients with AML secondary to MDS. The CR rate was 67% with an OS of 9 months and 5-year survival of 15%.[64] The FOSSIL study retrospectively analyzed patients with sAML who received either FLAG or 7 + 3; these data showed FLAG had a higher response rate defined as CR + CRi + morphologic leukemia-free survival (MLFS) of 70% versus 48% but no difference in OS.[65] A further study by the EORTC-GIMEMA AML-12 trial evaluated high-dose cytarabine in induction, with patients age 15 to 60 years receiving daunorubicin, etoposide and either cytarabine ($100 mg/m^2$ daily) for 10 days or high-dose cytarabine ($3000 mg/m^2$) twice daily on days 1, 3, 5, and 7. The high-dose cytarabine group achieved higher CR rates, particularly in patients under the age of 46 years, and subgroup analysis demonstrated an improvement in the CR rate in patients with sAML for younger (OR 5.99) and older (OR 3.75) patients.[66] Although intensive chemotherapy has induced some improved responses by changing agents, a retrospective analysis in 299 patients with high-risk MDS and sAML demonstrated that patients who received intensive chemotherapy did not have an improvement in overall survival compared with those not undergoing intensive chemotherapy.[67]

Hypomethylating Agents

Hypomethylating agents are often the backbone of sAML treatment due the simple fact that these patients are often older, have comorbidities, and are not eligible for induction chemotherapy. Treatment with the hypomethylating agents, decitabine and azacitidine, is effective in MDS and sAML patients, because these diseases have an abundance of DNA methylation.[68] In the AZA-001 study, which was a phase III study comparing azacitidine to conventional care, 34% of the patients were classified as having refractory anemia with excess blasts in transformation (RAEBT), now defined as AML. Although there were not subset data for these RAEBT patients, the study showed an overall improvement in the azacitidine arm with regards to OS compared with best supportive care (HR 0.58, P-=.0045), and time to transformation to AML across all subgroups (HR 0.50, P<.0001).[69] A French retrospective study evaluated azacitidine compared with IC in sAML and demonstrated no difference in OS (azacitidine 10.8 months, IC 9.6 months, P=.899). Subgroup analysis showed that in patients who had not received treatment in 1.6 years for their antecedent disease, the IC arm had a lower risk of death compared with azacitidine (HR 0.61, 95% confidence interval (CI) 0.38–0.99 at 1.6 years).[70]

Decitabine at the standard 5-day dose was also evaluated in a randomized phase III trial versus best supportive care or LDAC in older AML patients.[71] This study, which had 39.3% of participants defined as sAML, demonstrated a nonsignificant difference in median OS with decitabine, with HR in sAML also nonsignificant (0.92; 0.66–1.29).[71] Decitabine has recently undertaken a much more prominent role it the treatment of p53 AML. In a paper by Welch and colleagues,[72] 21 of 21 patients with TP53 mutations responded to 10-day decitabine at a dose of 20 mg/m^2 with a median response duration of 12.7 months. Although this paper did not specifically subset for AHD or tAML, the TP53 mutation alone is highly linked to these diagnoses.[7]

Novel Agents

Gemtuzumab ozogamicin (GO) is a humanized antibody-drug conjugate that binds an anti-CD33 immunoglobulin G_4 antibody to the DNA toxin calicheamicin. It received accelerated FDA approval in 2000 for CD33 + AML, but was voluntarily withdrawn in June 2010 after a postmarketing study demonstrated a higher induction mortality with no improvement in CR or RFS.[73] The drug was then reapproved in September 2017 based on new safety data with a lower fractionated dosing regimen.[74] This study showed an improvement at 2 years in EFS (40.8% vs 17.1%), OS (53.2% vs 41.9%) and RFS (50.3% vs 22.7%). In subset analysis, it appears that the favorable or intermediate-risk cytogenetic groups had the best responses. The study was not analyzed for sAML.

Further studies analyzed which patients would benefit most from the addition of gemtuzumab.[75] Again, results from this study favored the favorable cytogenetic group, with a trend for benefit in the intermediate-risk group, and no benefit for the poor-risk group. A further study specifically evaluated older patients from age 61 to 75 years, including an sAML subset (29.7%).[76] No subgroup had benefit from the addition of GO with regards to CR or OS, although a nonsignificant trend in the sAML for benefit was noted. A smaller trial attempted a different strategy by combining GO with arsenic trioxide in patients with sAML or MDS. This phase II study yielded a response in 30% of patients, with a median OS of 9.7 months.[77]

B-cell leukemia/lymphoma-2 (BCL2) is an antiapoptotic protein that promotes survival of leukemic blast through regulation of the mitochondrial apoptotic pathway. Sensitizer BCL-2 homology 3 (BH3) proteins are antagonists of these antiapoptotic proteins and therefore promote apoptosis via mitochondrial outer membrane permeabilization.[78] Venetoclax, an oral small molecule BCL-2 inhibitor, demonstrated on-target BCL-2 inhibition by BH3 profiling and an overall response rate of 19% in a single agent trial in very advanced AML.[79] Venetoclax was combined with HMA in a phase IB dose escalation and expansion study in an elderly, unfit population. This study resulted in a CR + CRi rate of 73% at that selected dose of venetoclax 400 mg daily. Although not a planned subset, the sAML population accounted for 25% of the study population and had the same CR + CRi rate as the de novo population, but potentially a longer duration of response (not reached [NR] vs 9.4 months) and OS (NR vs 12.5 months). These data led to the FDA approval of venetoclax in combination with HMA for the treatment of newly diagnosed AML in adults age 75 or older or who have comorbidities that preclude the use of intensive induction chemotherapy.

A second phase IB/II study combined venetoclax with low-dose cytarabine in a similar untreated AML population ineligible for intensive chemotherapy.[80] The CR + CRi rate with this regimen was 54%, with a recommended phase II dose of venetoclax at 600 mg daily. The sAML population comprised 49% of the study, with the CR + CRi rate markedly worse in the sAML population compared with the de novo population (35% vs 71%).

Bone Marrow Transplant Studies

It is common knowledge that sAML patients are rarely if ever cured with conventional chemotherapy, and therefore data from consolidative bone marrow or stem cell transplants (BMT) are imperative when discussing long-term prognosis. Early studies demonstrated a 2-year OS, EFS, relapse rate, and transplant-related mortality of 30%, 28%, 42%, and 49%, respectively.[81] More recent retrospective studies often combine MDS and sAML patients; 1 study demonstrates a 4-year estimate for OS of 31%, with multivariate analysis showing reduced intensity conditioning (RIC) transplants and advanced stage associated with increased relapse.[82] A second study showed OS of 37% at 1 year and 22% at 5 years, with multivariate analysis demonstrating age greater than 35, poor risk cytogenetics, t-AML or advanced t-MDS, and donor other than HLA identical sibling or partially or well-matched unrelated donor was associated with worsened DFS and OS.[83] A large retrospective study by the Acute Leukemia Working Party of the European Society for Blood and Bone Marrow Transplantation evaluated 4997 patients with sAML.[84] Two-year OS was 44.5%, and patients receiving myeloablative regimens had decreased relapse and higher non-relapse mortality, but no difference in OS from RIC regimens. Allogeneic transplant was associated with improved survival compared with no transplant in sAML patients, particularly those who had failed hypomethylating treatment.[85] However, despite the data establishing the poor prognosis of sAML, 2 separate retrospective studies demonstrated comparable outcomes between sAML and de novo AML in first remission.[86,87]

Further transplant variables may determine the outcome of sAML patients. Another European study by the Acute Leukemia Working Party evaluation transplants in sAML demonstrated myeloablative transplants yielded lower relapse rates and improved overall survival compared with RIC tranplants.[88] Furthermore, source of stems cells may also play a role in outcome; a retrospective study in sAML patients showed umbilical cord transplants were associated with higher risk of grade II-IV acute graft-versus-host disease compared with haploidentical transplants with no difference chronic GVHD, relapse rate, nonrelapse mortality, LFS, and OS.[89] Unfortunately, BMT is not always curative, and patients with sAML who relapse after transplant have a median survival rate of 4.7 months and a 2-year survival rate of only 17.7%.[90]

SUMMARY

The treatment of sAML has evolved from the singular option of standard 7 + 3 induction chemotherapy. Although the discovery of novel inhibitors such as the FLT3 inhibitors of IDH inhibitors has provided targeted therapy for all patients with AML, these agents do not provide the therapeutic boost to sAML patients, as these mutations are infrequent. However, advances in chemotherapy such as Vyxeos (liposomal daunorubicin:cytarabine) have proven overall benefit in sAML over 7 + 3 in fit candidates, and the addition of venetoclax to HMA in the unfit population seems to benefit both de novo and sAML. Furthermore, the treatment of prolonged decitabine dosing may benefit p53 mutant AML, which is a large component in the sAML population. As a better understanding of the molecular aspects of de novo AML and sAML is gained, the mutations and mechanisms of sAML should be better targeted, leading to improved efficacy and safety.

DISCLOSURE

Advisory Board: Jazz Pharmaceuticals, Pfizer Inc.

REFERENCES

1. Siegel RL, Miller KD, Jemal A. Cancer statistics, 2018. CA Cancer J Clin 2018; 68:7–30.
2. Winer ES, Stone RM. Novel therapy in acute myeloid leukemia (AML): moving toward targeted approaches. Ther Adv Hematol 2019;10. 2040620719860645.
3. National Cancer Institute. SEER cancer stat facts: acute myeloid leukemia (AML). Available at: https://seer.cancer.gov/statfacts/html/amyl.html/. Accessed December 17, 2018.
4. Leone G, Mele L, Pulsoni A, et al. The incidence of secondary leukemias. Haematologica 1999;84:937–45.
5. Østgård LSG, Medeiros BC, Sengeløv H, et al. Epidemiology and clinical significance of secondary and therapy-related acute myeloid leukemia: a national population-based cohort study. J Clin Oncol 2015;33:3641–9.
6. Arber DA, Orazi A, Hasserjian R, et al. The 2016 revision to the World Health Organization classification of myeloid neoplasms and acute leukemia. Blood 2016; 127:2391–405.
7. Lindsley RC, Mar BG, Mazzola E, et al. Acute myeloid leukemia ontogeny is defined by distinct somatic mutations. Blood 2015;125:1367–76.
8. Welch John S, Ley Timothy J, Link Daniel C, et al. The origin and evolution of mutations in acute myeloid leukemia. Cell 2012;150:264–78.
9. Vardiman JW, Thiele J, Arber DA, et al. The 2008 revision of the World Health Organization (WHO) classification of myeloid neoplasms and acute leukemia: rationale and important changes. Blood 2009;114:937–51.
10. Weinberg OK, Arber DA. Acute myeloid leukemia with myelodysplasia-related changes: a new definition. Surg Pathol Clin 2010;3:1153–64.
11. Devillier R, Gelsi-Boyer V, Brecqueville M, et al. Acute myeloid leukemia with myelodysplasia-related changes are characterized by a specific molecular pattern with high frequency of ASXL1 mutations. Am J Hematol 2012;87:659–62.

12. Devillier R, Mansat-De Mas V, Gelsi-Boyer V, et al. Role of ASXL1 and TP53 mutations in the molecular classification and prognosis of acute myeloid leukemias with myelodysplasia-related changes. Oncotarget 2015;6:8388–96.

13. Xu X-Q, Wang J-M, Gao L, et al. Characteristics of acute myeloid leukemia with myelodysplasia-related changes: a retrospective analysis in a cohort of Chinese patients. Am J Hematol 2014;89:874–81.

14. Ossenkoppele G, Montesinos P. Challenges in the diagnosis and treatment of secondary acute myeloid leukemia. Crit Rev Oncol Hematol 2019;138:6–13.

15. Bhatia S. Therapy-related myelodysplasia and acute myeloid leukemia. Semin Oncol 2013;40:666–75.

16. Cheung E, Perissinotti AJ, Bixby DL, et al. The leukemia strikes back: a review of pathogenesis and treatment of secondary AML. Ann Hematol 2019;98:541–59.

17. Leone G, Pagano L, Ben-Yehuda D, et al. Therapy-related leukemia and myelodysplasia: susceptibility and incidence. Haematologica 2007;92:1389–98.

18. Zhang W, Becciolini A, Biggeri A, et al. Second malignancies in breast cancer patients following radiotherapy: a study in Florence, Italy. Breast Cancer Res 2011; 13:R38.

19. Curtis RE, Boice JD, Stovall M, et al. Risk of leukemia after chemotherapy and radiation treatment for breast cancer. N Engl J Med 1992;326:1745–51.

20. Mauritzson N, Albin M, Rylander L, et al. Pooled analysis of clinical and cytogenetic features in treatment-related and de novo adult acute myeloid leukemia and myelodysplastic syndromes based on a consecutive series of 761 patients analyzed 1976–1993 and on 5098 unselected cases reported in the literature 1974–2001. Leukemia 2002;16:2366–78.

21. Pedersen-Bjergaard J, Andersen MK, Andersen MT, et al. Genetics of therapy-related myelodysplasia and acute myeloid leukemia. Leukemia 2008;22:240.

22. Olney HJ, Mitelman F, Johansson B, et al. Unique balanced chromosome abnormalities in treatment-related myelodysplastic syndromes and acute myeloid leukemia: report from an International Workshop. Genes Chromosomes Cancer 2002;33:413–23.

23. Schoch C, Kern W, Schnittger S, et al. Karyotype is an independent prognostic parameter in therapy-related acute myeloid leukemia (t-AML): an analysis of 93 patients with t-AML in comparison to 1091 patients with de novo AML. Leukemia 2004;18:120–5.

24. Ok CY, Patel KP, Garcia-Manero G, et al. TP53 mutation characteristics in therapy-related myelodysplastic syndromes and acute myeloid leukemia is similar to de novo diseases. J Hematol Oncol 2015;8:45.

25. Rücker FG, Schlenk RF, Bullinger L, et al. TP53 alterations in acute myeloid leukemia with complex karyotype correlate with specific copy number alterations, monosomal karyotype, and dismal outcome. Blood 2012;119:2114–21.

26. Kadia TM, Jain P, Ravandi F, et al. TP53 mutations in newly diagnosed acute myeloid leukemia: clinicomolecular characteristics, response to therapy, and outcomes. Cancer 2016;122(22):3484–91.

27. Jaiswal S, Fontanillas P, Flannick J, et al. Age-related clonal hematopoiesis associated with adverse outcomes. N Engl J Med 2014;371:2488–98.

28. Wong TN, Ramsingh G, Young AL, et al. Role of TP53 mutations in the origin and evolution of therapy-related acute myeloid leukaemia. Nature 2014;518:552.

29. Yoshizato T, Dumitriu B, Hosokawa K, et al. Somatic mutations and clonal hematopoiesis in aplastic anemia. N Engl J Med 2015;373:35–47.

30. Germing U, Strupp C, Kuendgen A, et al. Prospective validation of the WHO proposals for the classification of myelodysplastic syndromes. Haematologica 2006; 91:1596–604.

31. Walter MJ, Shen D, Ding L, et al. Clonal architecture of secondary acute myeloid leukemia. N Engl J Med 2012;366:1090–8.

32. Flach J, Dicker F, Schnittger S, et al. An accumulation of cytogenetic and molecular genetic events characterizes the progression from MDS to secondary AML: an analysis of 38 paired samples analyzed by cytogenetics, molecular mutation analysis and SNP microarray profiling. Leukemia 2011;25:713.

33. Takahashi K, Jabbour E, Wang X, et al. Dynamic acquisition of FLT3 or RAS alterations drive a subset of patients with lower risk MDS to secondary AML. Leukemia 2013;27:2081.

34. Sperling AS, Gibson CJ, Ebert BL. The genetics of myelodysplastic syndrome: from clonal haematopoiesis to secondary leukaemia. Nat Rev Cancer 2016;17:5.

35. Dicker F, Haferlach C, Sundermann J, et al. Mutation analysis for RUNX1, MLL-PTD, FLT3-ITD, NPM1 and NRAS in 269 patients with MDS or secondary AML. Leukemia 2010;24:1528.

36. Tsai S-C, Shih L-Y, Liang S-T, et al. Biological activities of RUNX1 mutants predict secondary acute leukemia transformation from chronic myelomonocytic leukemia and myelodysplastic syndromes. Clin Cancer Res 2015;21:3541–51.

37. Fried I, Bodner C, Pichler MM, et al. Frequency, onset and clinical impact of somatic DNMT3A mutations in therapy-related and secondary acute myeloid leukemia. Haematologica 2012;97:246–50.

38. Shukron O, Vainstein V, Kündgen A, et al. Analyzing transformation of myelodysplastic syndrome to secondary acute myeloid leukemia using a large patient database. Am J Hematol 2012;87:853–60.

39. Milosevic JD, Puda A, Malcovati L, et al. Clinical significance of genetic aberrations in secondary acute myeloid leukemia. Am J Hematol 2012;87:1010–6.

40. Aynardi J, Manur R, Hess PR, et al. JAK2 V617F-positive acute myeloid leukaemia (AML): a comparison between de novo AML and secondary AML transformed from an underlying myeloproliferative neoplasm. A study from the Bone Marrow Pathology Group. Br J Haematol 2018;182:78–85.

41. Rampal R, Ahn J, Abdel-Wahab O, et al. Genomic and functional analysis of leukemic transformation of myeloproliferative neoplasms. Proc Natl Acad Sci U S A 2014;111:E5401–10.

42. Poynter JN, Richardson M, Roesler M, et al. Chemical exposures and risk of acute myeloid leukemia and myelodysplastic syndromes in a population-based study. Int J Cancer 2017;140:23–33.

43. Ertz-Archambault N, Kosiorek H, Taylor GE, et al. Association of therapy for autoimmune disease with myelodysplastic syndromes and acute myeloid leukemia. JAMA Oncol 2017;3:936–43.

44. Ge I, Saliba RM, Maadani F, et al. Patient age and number of apheresis days may predict development of secondary myelodysplastic syndrome and acute myelogenous leukemia after high-dose chemotherapy and autologous stem cell transplantation for lymphoma. Transfusion 2017;57:1052–7.

45. Hulegårdh E, Nilsson C, Lazarevic V, et al. Characterization and prognostic features of secondary acute myeloid leukemia in a population-based setting: a report from the Swedish Acute Leukemia Registry. Am J Hematol 2015;90:208–14.

46. Kayser S, Döhner K, Krauter J, et al. The impact of therapy-related acute myeloid leukemia (AML) on outcome in 2853 adult patients with newly diagnosed AML. Blood 2011;117:2137–45.

47. Szotkowski T, Muzik J, Voglova J, et al. Prognostic factors and treatment outcome in 1,516 adult patients with de novo and secondary acute myeloid leukemia in 1999–2009 in 5 hematology intensive care centers in the Czech Republic. Neoplasia 2010;57:578–89.

48. Schetelig J, de Wreede LC, van Gelder M, et al. Late treatment-related mortality versus competing causes of death after allogeneic transplantation for myelodysplastic syndromes and secondary acute myeloid leukemia. Leukemia 2019;33: 686–95.

49. Rizzieri DA, O'Brien JA, Broadwater G, et al. Outcomes of patients who undergo aggressive induction therapy for secondary acute myeloid leukemia. Cancer 2009;115:2922–9.

50. Boddu P, Kantarjian HM, Garcia-Manero G, et al. Treated secondary acute myeloid leukemia: a distinct high-risk subset of AML with adverse prognosis. Blood Adv 2017;1:1312–23.

51. Boddu PC, Kantarjian HM, Ravandi F, et al. Characteristics and outcomes of older patients with secondary acute myeloid leukemia according to treatment approach. Cancer 2017;123:3050–60.

52. Bertoli S, Tavitian S, Bories P, et al. Outcome of patients aged 60-75 years with newly diagnosed secondary acute myeloid leukemia: a single-institution experience. Cancer Med 2019;8(8):3846–54.

53. Stölzel F, Pfirrmann M, Aulitzky WE, et al. Risk stratification using a new prognostic score for patients with secondary acute myeloid leukemia: results of the prospective AML96 trial. Leukemia 2010;25:420.

54. Yates JW, Wallace HJ, Ellison RR, et al. Cytosine arabinoside (NSC-63878) and daunorubicin (NSC-83142) therapy in acute nonlymphocytic leukemia. Cancer Chemother Rep 1973;57:485–8.

55. Lee J-H, Joo Y-D, Kim H, et al. A randomized trial comparing standard versus high-dose daunorubicin induction in patients with acute myeloid leukemia. Blood 2011;118:3832–41.

56. Fernandez HF, Sun Z, Yao X, et al. Anthracycline dose intensification in acute myeloid leukemia. N Engl J Med 2009;361:1249–59.

57. Lowenberg B, Ossenkoppele GJ, van Putten W, et al. High-dose daunorubicin in older patients with acute myeloid leukemia. N Engl J Med 2009;361:1235–48.

58. Burnett AK, Russell NH, Hills RK, et al. A randomized comparison of daunorubicin 90 mg/m2 vs 60 mg/m2 in AML induction: results from the UK NCRI AML17 trial in 1206 patients. Blood 2015;125:3878–85.

59. Feldman EJ, Kolitz JE, Trang JM, et al. Pharmacokinetics of CPX-351; a nanoscale liposomal fixed molar ratio formulation of cytarabine:daunorubicin, in patients with advanced leukemia. Leuk Res 2012;36:1283–9.

60. Feldman EJ, Lancet JE, Kolitz JE, et al. First-in-man study of CPX-351: a liposomal carrier containing cytarabine and daunorubicin in a fixed 5:1 molar ratio for the treatment of relapsed and refractory acute myeloid leukemia. J Clin Oncol 2011;29:979–85.

61. Lancet JE, Cortes JE, Hogge DE, et al. Phase 2 trial of CPX-351, a fixed 5:1 molar ratio of cytarabine/daunorubicin, vs cytarabine/daunorubicin in older adults with untreated AML. Blood 2014;123:3239–46.

62. Lancet JE, Uy GL, Cortes JE, et al. CPX-351 (cytarabine and daunorubicin) liposome for injection versus conventional cytarabine plus daunorubicin in older

patients with newly diagnosed secondary acute myeloid leukemia. J Clin Oncol 2018;36:2684–92.

63. Walter RB, Othus M, Orlowski KF, et al. Unsatisfactory efficacy in randomized study of reduced-dose CPX-351 for medically less fit adults with newly diagnosed acute myeloid leukemia or other high-grade myeloid neoplasm. Haematologica 2018;103:e106–9.

64. Ferrara F, Palmieri S, Izzo T, et al. Continuous sequential infusion of fludarabine and cytarabine for elderly patients with acute myeloid leukaemia secondary to a previously diagnosed myelodysplastic syndrome. Hematol Oncol 2010;28: 202–8.

65. Vulaj V, Perissinotti AJ, Uebel JR, et al. The FOSSIL Study: FLAG or standard 7+3 induction therapy in secondary acute myeloid leukemia. Leuk Res 2018;70:91–6.

66. Willemze R, Suciu S, Meloni G, et al. High-dose cytarabine in induction treatment improves the outcome of adult patients younger than age 46 years with acute myeloid leukemia: results of the EORTC-GIMEMA AML-12 trial. J Clin Oncol 2013;32:219–28.

67. Schuler E, Zadrozny N, Blum S, et al. Long-term outcome of high risk patients with myelodysplastic syndromes or secondary acute myeloid leukemia receiving intensive chemotherapy. Ann Hematol 2018;97:2325–32.

68. Figueroa ME, Skrabanek L, Li Y, et al. MDS and secondary AML display unique patterns and abundance of aberrant DNA methylation. Blood 2009;114:3448–58.

69. Fenaux P, Mufti GJ, Hellstrom-Lindberg E, et al. Efficacy of azacitidine compared with that of conventional care regimens in the treatment of higher-risk myelodysplastic syndromes: a randomised, open-label, phase III study. Lancet Oncol 2009;10:223–32.

70. Dumas P-Y, Bertoli S, Bérard E, et al. Azacitidine or intensive chemotherapy for older patients with secondary or therapy-related acute myeloid leukemia. Oncotarget 2017;8:79126–36.

71. Kantarjian HM, Thomas XG, Dmoszynska A, et al. Multicenter, randomized, open-label, phase III trial of decitabine versus patient choice, with physician advice, of either supportive care or low-dose cytarabine for the treatment of older patients with newly diagnosed acute myeloid leukemia. J Clin Oncol 2012;30:2670–7.

72. Welch JS, Petti AA, Miller CA, et al. TP53 and decitabine in acute myeloid leukemia and myelodysplastic syndromes. N Engl J Med 2016;375:2023–36.

73. Wei AH, Tiong IS. Midostaurin, enasidenib, CPX-351, gemtuzumab ozogamicin, and venetoclax bring new hope to AML. Blood 2017;130:2469–74.

74. Castaigne S, Pautas C, Terré C, et al. Effect of gemtuzumab ozogamicin on survival of adult patients with de-novo acute myeloid leukaemia (ALFA-0701): a randomised, open-label, phase 3 study. Lancet 2012;379:1508–16.

75. Burnett AK, Hills RK, Milligan D, et al. Identification of patients with acute myeloblastic leukemia who benefit from the addition of gemtuzumab ozogamicin: results of the MRC AML15 trial. J Clin Oncol 2011;29:369–77.

76. Amadori S, Suciu S, Stasi R, et al. Sequential combination of gemtuzumab ozogamicin and standard chemotherapy in older patients with newly diagnosed acute myeloid leukemia: results of a randomized phase III trial by the EORTC and GIMEMA Consortium (AML-17). J Clin Oncol 2013;31:4424–30.

77. Sekeres MA, Maciejewski JP, Erba HP, et al. A Phase 2 study of combination therapy with arsenic trioxide and gemtuzumab ozogamicin in patients with myelodysplastic syndromes or secondary acute myeloid leukemia. Cancer 2011;117: 1253–61.

78. Konopleva M, Letai A. BCL-2 inhibition in AML - an unexpected bonus? Blood 2018;132(10):1007–12.
79. Konopleva M, Pollyea DA, Potluri J, et al. Efficacy and biological correlates of response in a phase II study of venetoclax monotherapy in patients with acute myelogenous leukemia. Crit Rev Oncol Hematol 2016;6:1106–17.
80. Wei AH Jr, Strickland SA, Hou J-Z, et al. Venetoclax combined with low-dose cytarabine for previously untreated patients with acute myeloid leukemia: results from a phase Ib/II study. J Clin Oncol 2019;37:1277–84.
81. Yakoub-Agha I, Salmonière PdL, Ribaud P, et al. Allogeneic bone marrow transplantation for therapy-related myelodysplastic syndrome and acute myeloid leukemia: a long-term study of 70 patients—report of the French Society of Bone Marrow Transplantation. J Clin Oncol 2000;18:963.
82. Lim Z, Brand R, Martino R, et al. Allogeneic hematopoietic stem-cell transplantation for patients 50 years or older with myelodysplastic syndromes or secondary acute myeloid leukemia. J Clin Oncol 2010;28:405–11.
83. Litzow MR, Tarima S, Pérez WS, et al. Allogeneic transplantation for therapy-related myelodysplastic syndrome and acute myeloid leukemia. Blood 2010; 115:1850–7.
84. Sengsayadeth S, Labopin M, Boumendil A, et al. Transplant outcomes for secondary acute myeloid leukemia: acute leukemia working party of the European Society for Blood and Bone Marrow Transplantation study. Biol Blood Marrow Transplant 2018;24:1406–14.
85. Shin SH, Yahng SA, Yoon JH, et al. Survival benefits with transplantation in secondary AML evolving from myelodysplastic syndrome with hypomethylating treatment failure. Bone Marrow Transplant 2012;48:678.
86. Michelis FV, Atenafu EG, Gupta V, et al. Comparable outcomes post allogeneic hematopoietic cell transplant for patients with de novo or secondary acute myeloid leukemia in first remission. Bone Marrow Transplant 2015;50:907.
87. Tang F-F, Huang X-J, Zhang X-H, et al. Allogeneic hematopoietic cell transplantation for adult patients with treatment-related acute myeloid leukemia during first remission: comparable to de novo acute myeloid leukemia. Leuk Res 2016; 47:8–15.
88. Sengsayadeth S, Gatwood KS, Boumendil A, et al. Conditioning intensity in secondary AML with prior myelodysplastic syndrome/myeloproliferative disorders: an EBMT ALWP study. Blood Adv 2018;2:2127–35.
89. Ruggeri A, Labopin M, Savani B, et al. Hematopoietic stem cell transplantation with unrelated cord blood or haploidentical donor grafts in adult patients with secondary acute myeloid leukemia, a comparative study from Eurocord and the ALWP EBMT. Bone Marrow Transplant 2019;54(12):1987–94.
90. Schmid C, de Wreede LC, van Biezen A, et al. Outcome after relapse of myelodysplastic syndrome and secondary acute myeloid leukemia following allogeneic stem cell transplantation: a retrospective registry analysis on 698 patients by the Chronic Malignancies Working Party of the European Society of Blood and Marrow Transplantation. Haematologica 2018;103:237–45.

Do Recent Randomized Trial Results Influence which Patients with Myelodysplastic Syndromes Receive Iron Chelation?

Norbert Gattermann, MD

KEYWORDS

- Myelodysplastic syndromes • Transfusion therapy • Iron overload • Iron chelation
- Deferasirox • Telesto trial

KEY POINTS

- There is no reason to believe that iron overload (IOL) is less toxic in elderly patients with myelodysplastic syndrome (MDS) than in young thalassemia patients. However, the impact of IOL is more difficult to prove in MDS, because of overlap with age-related clinical problems.
- Age-related comorbidities, particularly cardiovascular comorbidities, can increase the vulnerability to toxic effects of IOL in patients with MDS.
- In recent years, registry studies have consistently shown a survival benefit of iron chelation therapy (ICT) in patients with lower-risk MDS. These results are now corroborated by the improved event-free survival demonstrated by the Telesto study.
- ICT should be used in patients with transfusion-dependent MDS with a life expectancy of more than 2 years, perhaps including patients with higher-risk MDS responding to hypomethylating agents.

INTRODUCTION

Although iron is essential for a variety of pivotal biological processes, it can also be toxic. As it easily switches between its divalent (ferrous) and trivalent (ferric) form by accepting or losing an electron, iron is a strong catalyst for certain biochemical reactions, like the Fenton reaction, which generate reactive oxygen species. The latter are capable of attacking macromolecules and organelles, thereby causing cellular damage that eventually leads to tissue and organ dysfunction. This potential for toxicity

Department of Hematology, Oncology and Clinical Immunology, Heinrich Heine University Düsseldorf, Moorenstr. 5, Düsseldorf 40225, Germany
E-mail address: gattermann@med.uni-duesseldorf.de

Hematol Oncol Clin N Am 34 (2020) 465–473
https://doi.org/10.1016/j.hoc.2019.10.006
0889-8588/20/© 2019 Elsevier Inc. All rights reserved.

hemonc.theclinics.com

is increased by iron *overload* (IOL), which can result from inborn errors of metabolism, that is, various forms of hereditary hemochromatosis, and from chronic transfusion therapy. Every unit of packed red cells contains 200 to 250 mg of iron, whereas normal daily iron uptake in the duodenum is only 1 to 2 mg under steady state conditions. There is no physiologic mechanism for excreting surplus iron.

In the pre-chelation era, transfusional IOL was lethal for patients with beta-thalassemia major, who died as children or adolescents from intractable heart failure due to cardiac IOL. Iron *chelation* has an opposite effect. The striking improvement in survival of patients with transfusion-dependent thalassemia seen over the past 50 years reflects the availability of deferoxamine and other iron chelators for the treatment of IOL and the extent of patient compliance with treatment. In contrast to thalassemia major, the role of iron chelation therapy (ICT) in myelodysplastic syndromes (MDS) is less well defined and has been somewhat controversial.

IMPACT OF IRON OVERLOAD IN MYELODYSPLASTIC SYNDROME

Why is it difficult to extrapolate the knowledge from thalassemia into MDS, where IOL should have similar toxicity? First, exposure to IOL is usually shorter in MDS because transfusion therapy starts much later in life. Accordingly, many patients may not live long enough to develop clinical complications of IOL. Second, iron-related complications in elderly patients with MDS overlap with age-related medical problems. Even if iron-related complications add up to constitute a strong risk factor, this effect may easily hide behind the common causes of death in the elderly. It is therefore difficult to determine to what extent IOL contributes to morbidity and mortality in elderly patients with MDS. However, that does not mean that iron-related problems do not exist.

In fact, serum ferritin above a threshold of 1000 ng/mL has a clear dose-dependent impact on overall survival (OS) of patients with low risk MDS. Malcovati and colleagues[1] also demonstrated that serum ferritin is an *independent* prognostic factor in MDS, even if transfusion burden, which reflects the degree of bone marrow failure, is taken into account on multivariate analysis. Similarly, data from the European LeukemiaNet prospective MDS registry showed that besides transfusion burden, which was the most important prognostic factor, increasing levels of serum ferritin also had independent impact on OS of transfusion-dependent patients with lower-risk MDS. The same registry recently found survival rates to be inferior when labile plasma iron was detectable in patients with lower-risk MDS, whether the patients were transfusion-dependent or not.[2] This analysis has recently been updated with a larger number of patients, confirming that transfusion dependency is associated with the presence of toxic iron species and inferior survival.[3]

On the one hand, transfusion dependency predicts shortened survival because it reflects hematopoietic insufficiency, with all its possible complications, like infection, bleeding, and the detrimental effects of chronic anemia. On the other hand, transfusion dependency causes IOL, thereby creating a new medical problem that has its own negative impact on OS (**Fig. 1**).

Within that conceptual framework, cardiac dysfunction plays an important role, partly as a consequence of chronic anemia, partly as a consequence of age-related cardiac comorbidities, and partly as a consequence of IOL. Focusing on cardiac problems is justified because the heart is more vulnerable to IOL than the liver, and clinically relevant cardiac dysfunction occurs at much lower tissue iron concentrations than clinically relevant liver dysfunction.[4]

Besides cardiac damage, endothelial dysfunction is another iron-related clinical problem, which may have been underestimated so far. Macrophages in the vessel

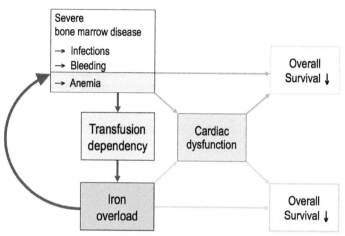

Fig. 1. Possible relationship among bone marrow failure, IOL, and prognosis in patients with MDS.

wall can accumulate iron from increased destruction of red blood cells (RBCs) or from disturbed iron homeostasis under the influence of hepcidin. When they accumulate iron, macrophages produce more reactive oxygen species and also show decreased efflux of cholesterol. The ensuing oxidative stress and cholesterol accumulation favor progression to foam cells and promote inflammation and apoptosis, eventually leading to plaque destabilization. Vinchi and colleagues[5] summarized the problem as follows: with increasing age, high circulating iron levels strongly enhance the severity of the atherosclerotic phenotype, indicating that systemic IOL is a risk factor for atherosclerosis progression and predisposes to cardiovascular disease.

This would imply that iron chelation may be beneficial in this context. Indeed, iron chelation was shown to improve endothelial function in patients with coronary artery disease. Deferoxamine improved nitric-oxide–mediated, endothelium-dependent vasodilation in patients with coronary artery disease, suggesting that iron availability contributes to impaired nitric oxide action in atherosclerosis.[6] A beneficial effect of ICT on arterial function was also demonstrated in patients with beta-thalassemia major.[7] Twelve months of iron chelation resulted in a significantly improved brachial artery flow–mediated dilation and significantly decreased carotid arterial stiffness index. This was ascribed to the ability of deferasirox (DFX) to bind labile cellular iron pools in the vascular wall, thus diminishing reactive oxygen species formation and attenuating nitric oxide inactivation.

Increased risk of infection is another clinical problem related to IOL. Canadian investigators recently performed a retrospective analysis for lower-risk patients with MDS receiving RBC transfusions and observed that receiving ICT was associated with superior OS. Although number and type of infections were similar between groups, and despite similar neutrophil counts, time to first infection was significantly longer in patients receiving ICT.[8] These results should be confirmed in larger, prospective analyses.

Regarding iron-related organ damage, the bone marrow should be reckoned among the organs that suffer from IOL. IOL may aggravate bone marrow dysfunction in MDS and may thus set up a vicious cycle (see **Fig. 1**). With respect to the hematopoietic system, 2 scenarios of IOL should be distinguished. On the one hand, IOL in hereditary hemochromatosis and thalassemia major occurs in the context of a polyclonal nonmalignant bone marrow with sufficient antioxidative defenses and DNA repair, and therefore does not lead to substantial bone marrow dysfunction. On the other hand, IOL in MDS puts additional strain on a clonally transformed, premalignant bone marrow, where oxidative stress is already increased and antioxidative defenses and DNA repair seem to be insufficient to prevent iron-related aggravation of bone marrow dysfunction. A number of case reports, small patient series, and larger studies have shown that ICT can improve hematopoiesis in a proportion of patients with MDS.[9]

SURVIVAL IMPACT OF IRON CHELATION THERAPY IN MYELODYSPLASTIC SYNDROME

In view of several potential benefits of ICT, the question arises whether these benefits translate into improved OS. Multiple studies consistently suggested that ICT significantly improves OS in patients with transfusion-dependent MDS. The main problem with these retrospective studies is that patient populations were usually well characterized regarding disease-related parameters and risk factors, but not characterized and stratified according to overall performance status. This may have biased the results because younger, fitter patients may have been more likely to receive iron chelation, thereby inflating the benefit of ICT. Two registry studies went to great lengths to avoid such bias. One is from the Canadian MDS Registry, which carefully documents performance status and comorbidities. A significant survival benefit of ICT was found when roughly comparable cohorts were analyzed, and this was further corroborated by applying several important matching criteria.[10] Another thorough analysis was conducted in the prospective European LeukemiaNet MDS (EUMDS) Registry, which similarly adjusted for relevant prognostic factors and also ascertained a significant survival benefit of ICT.[11] All the registry data point in the same direction, implying a survival advantage of ICT in lower-risk MDS, and the quality of at least 2 of the registry studies has improved to a point where it becomes hard to ignore the survival benefit of iron chelation.

A RANDOMIZED, PLACEBO-CONTROLLED CLINICAL TRIAL OF IRON CHELATION THERAPY IN MYELODYSPLASTIC SYNDROME

Despite mounting evidence from registry studies, many hematologists have been waiting for results from a prospective placebo-controlled clinical trial of ICT in MDS. The only such trial is the Telesto study, which was presented at the American Society of Hematology meeting in 2018.[12] Telesto was initially designed as a phase III trial with a target enrollment of 630 patients. As a result of enrollment issues in countries in which deferasirox is licensed and reimbursed, the target sample size was reduced to 210 patients, based on the feasibility of enrolling patients and consultations with the health authorities. Between April 22, 2010, and February 2, 2015, 225 patients were included in 60 centers across 16 countries. Patients were randomized 2:1 to deferasirox (n = 149) or placebo (n = 76) and received study treatment from 10 to 40 mg/kg per day based on dosing guidelines. Participants had to have lower-risk MDS with a transfusion history of 15 to 75 packed red blood cells units and a serum ferritin (SF) >1000 ng/mL. They were not allowed to have a history of hospitalization due to congestive heart failure, and had to have a left ventricular ejection fraction above 50%. Substantial preexisting liver problems or kidney injury were also considered key exclusion criteria.

The primary endpoint of the study was event-free survival (EFS), which was measured using a composite primary endpoint of time from randomization to time of first documented nonfatal event (related to cardiac and liver function and transformation to acute myelogenous leukemia [AML]) or death, whichever occurred first. For example, if a patient developed worsening cardiac function and was sequentially hospitalized for congestive heart failure, and both were confirmed by the external adjudicating committee (EAC), only the first occurring event was counted as primary endpoint met. Nonfatal events were worsening cardiac function, hospitalization for congestive heart failure, liver function impairment, liver cirrhosis, and transformation into AML. Events were reviewed and confirmed by an independent adjudication committee.

Key secondary endpoints were OS, change in SF level, hematologic improvement in terms of erythroid response (based on International MDS Working Group criteria), change in endocrine function (thyroid and glycemic control), and safety. As the sample size did not provide sufficient power to test statistical hypotheses, all statistical tests performed were exploratory.

Key demographic and baseline characteristics were very similar in the DFX arm and the placebo arm of the study. Of note, the proportion of patients older than 75 years was larger in the DFX arm. At the time of data cutoff (April 28, 2018), all patients had discontinued from the study. Looking at primary reasons for end of treatment, more patients in the DFX arm than the placebo arm went off study because of adverse events (AEs), mainly increases in creatinine. Interestingly, more patients in the placebo arm discontinued by their own or by guardian decision. This was mainly because of a lack in decrease of SF levels. The median time on treatment was longer with DFX than with placebo (587.5 vs 370.5 days, respectively), and 43.9% and 25.0% of DFX and placebo patients, respectively, received treatment for ≥ 2 years. Most patients in the placebo arm (51.3%) were treated for less than 1 year; 5.4% of patients in the DFX arm were treated for 5 years or more (0% in placebo). The mean dose was lower with DFX (14.9 mg/kg per day) than with placebo (23.5 mg/kg per day), reflecting dose adjustments for changes in SF level. As expected, only patients on DFX achieved a decrease and stabilization of SF levels.

The most common ($\geq 15\%$) exposure-adjusted AEs with DFX and placebo, respectively, were diarrhea (24.7 vs 23.9%), pyrexia (21.8 vs 18.7%), increased blood creatinine (15.9 vs 0.9%), and upper respiratory tract infection (16.7 vs 22.7%). The only AE that occurred significantly more frequently with DFX was an increase in serum creatinine. This is a well-known side effect of DFX. Patients often develop a 25% increase in creatinine soon after start of treatment and then reach a plateau. However, some older patients with MDS must discontinue treatment because of further increases in serum creatinine.

Regarding the primary study endpoint of EFS, predefined events occurred in 49% of patients on placebo and 42% of patients on DFX. Median time to event was 1091 days in the placebo arm and 1440 days in the DFX arm. The difference was almost exactly 1 year, which corresponds to a 36.4% risk reduction in the DFX arm.

The Kaplan-Meier curves for EFS with DFX and placebo separate after approximately 2 years, which is plausible because it takes time for iron-related organ damage to develop, and therefore also takes time until the clinical benefit of ICT can manifest itself.

Regarding predefined nonfatal events that occurred first as confirmed by the adjudicating committee, the clearest difference between DFX-treated and placebo-treated patients was observed in terms of cardiac problems. Worsening of cardiac function and hospitalization for congestive heart failure occurred in a smaller proportion of DFX-treated patients. Although Telesto was not powered to detect differences between DFX and placebo for single-event categories of the composite primary endpoint for EFS, results are consistent with the view that cardiac dysfunction is an important component of the negative survival impact of IOL in elderly patients with MDS.

DFX treatment yielded superior EFS across all patient subgroups of clinical interest. It is noteworthy that patients older than 65 derived greater benefit than younger patients. This may suggest that older patients have more comorbidities, which renders them more vulnerable to the toxic effects of IOL and thus more likely to benefit from ICT.

Regarding OS, Kaplan-Meier curves are superimposable before they separate after approximately 5 years. However, as in many placebo-controlled trials, a proportion of patients on the placebo arm received the verum treatment after study drug discontinuation. In the Telesto study, 52% of placebo patients started ICT after study drug discontinuation. This may have shrouded any survival benefit of DFX in the comparison. The investigators of the study conclude that Telesto provides evidence on the clinical benefit of ICT in lower-risk patients with MDS with IOL.

HOW DOES THE TELESTO DATA CHANGE OUR CURRENT UNDERSTANDING OF THE ROLE OF IRON CHELATION THERAPY IN PATIENTS WITH TRANSFUSION-DEPENDENT LOWER-RISK MYELODYSPLASTIC SYNDROME WITH IRON OVERLOAD?

For the "believers" in ICT, this randomized clinical trial does not really change anything. Instead, it implies that the believers have always been right. The results will thus be appreciated as clearly supporting the use of ICT in transfusion-dependent patients with lower-risk MDS. On the other hand, the "nonbelievers" may still not be convinced and may argue that the study, after reduction of the sample size by two-thirds, did not have enough statistical power to provide irrefutable evidence of a substantial benefit of ICT. A certain degree of uncertainty will thus persist because, considering the current treatment landscape, it is unlikely that a similar randomized trial will be performed.

WHICH RESULTS IN PARTICULAR ARE NOVEL AND POTENTIALLY CLINICALLY MEANINGFUL?

A meaningful result of the Telesto study was the 1-year increase in EFS. However, as the trial was not powered to detect differences between DFX and placebo for single-event categories of the composite primary endpoint for EFS, it is not clear how the benefit can be attributed to specific causes. The data suggest that a decrease in cardiac complications may have been the most important contributor. The Kaplan-Meier curves for EFS separate after approximately 2 years, which is compatible with the fact that iron-related cardiac problems develop slowly. Accordingly, it takes some time until the benefit of ICT can manifest itself.

Corroborating the Telesto data, a Canadian retrospective analysis recently showed that for patients with transfusion-dependent lower-risk MDS, time to first cardiac event (TTCE) following RBC transfusion dependency was significantly longer in patients receiving ICT. On multivariate analysis, receiving ICT was an independent predictor for TTCE and OS.[13] Previously, a Spanish study had also demonstrated by multivariate analysis that iron chelation was a predictor for cardiac EFS ($P = .040$).[14] These results suggest that ICT may delay cardiac events in transfused patients.

DO THE STUDY RESULTS AFFECT ELIGIBILITY, TIMING, AND GOALS FOR IRON CHELATION THERAPY?

Regarding eligibility, the EFS benefit achieved after 2 years of treatment suggests that patients with transfusion-dependent MDS with a life expectancy of more than 2 years should receive ICT. Although the Telesto study included only patients with lower-risk MDS, this recommendation may extend to patients with higher-risk MDS who show a good response to hypomethylating agents and thus may experience improved survival.

As to the timing of ICT, the increase in EFS in the Telesto trial was achieved in patients with an SF above 1000 ng/mL, thus validating current guidelines recommending ICT in patients with an SF $\geq$1000 ng/mL. The effect in patients with lower SF levels has not been tested in this trial. It is an open question whether ICT therapy should be started earlier, considering that, besides achieving a negative iron balance, permanent suppression of iron-related oxidative stress is a major goal of ICT.

DO THE DATA PRESENT ANY NEW OR UNEXPECTED ADVERSE EVENTS COMPARED WITH CURRENT MEDICAL PRACTICE?

In the Telesto trial, the incidence rate of diarrhea during DFX treatment, which was a matter of concern in previous trials with patients with MDS, was no longer increased over that in the placebo arm. Apparently, physicians have learned how to manage this problem, partly with the help of guidelines providing therapeutic algorithms. In addition, it looks as if most physicians no longer use the recommended starting dose of DFX but initiate treatment with half the recommended dose.

The only AE in the Telesto trial that was significantly more common in patients receiving ICT therapy was an increase in serum creatine. Increased blood creatinine during DFX treatment had an incidence rate of 16 per 100 subject treatment years, which was 16 times higher than in the placebo arm. Elderly patients with MDS are more susceptible to renal impairment during ICT than young patients with thalassemia. Nevertheless, it is interesting to take note of a study on renal dysfunction in beta-thalassemia patients, which was based on the rationale that dose-dependent increases of serum creatinine levels during DFX treatment are attributable to changes in intraglomerular hemodynamics.[15] Piga and colleagues[16] studied the long-term effect of DFX 30 mg/kg per day on glomerular filtration rate (GFR) and renal plasma flow (RPF). The study included 2 washout periods, at weeks 8 to 10 and weeks 104 to 108. DFX influenced renal hemodynamics, reflected by a decrease in RPF, leading to a decrease in GFR. These effects were reversible after drug interruption over the short-term and long-term. Serum creatinine and creatinine clearance followed a similar pattern. Effects of DFX on renal hemodynamics were mild and reversible for up to 2 years of treatment, with no progressive worsening of renal function over time. Although these results are reassuring, there is a lack of corresponding data for older patients with MDS, who often have additional age-related renal dysfunction, sometimes leading to intolerability of ICT.

WHAT TYPE OF ADDITIONAL STUDIES COULD BE USEFUL TO FURTHER EVALUATE THE ROLE OF IRON CHELATION THERAPY IN PATIENTS WITH TRANSFUSION-DEPENDENT LOW/INTERMEDIATE-1 RISK MYELODYSPLASTIC SYNDROME WITH IRON OVERLOAD?

As already mentioned, it is an open question whether ICT should be started much earlier than current guidelines suggest. Such an approach may be beneficial and easy to implement because it would allow substantially lower doses of iron chelation to be used, which are well tolerated and, as recent research has shown for DFX, seem to be particularly suited to exert beneficial effects on erythroid precursor cells.[17] A clinical trial testing this approach is now being conducted in France.

SUMMARY

IOL is probably as toxic in elderly patients with MDS as it is in young patients with thalassemia, but the impact of IOL is more difficult to prove in MDS, because of the overlap between iron-related and age-related clinical problems. It is reasonable to assume that age-related comorbidities increase patients' vulnerability to the toxic effects of IOL, and that cardiovascular dysfunction, aggravated by IOL, is particularly relevant in elderly patients with MDS. Iron chelation can help to avoid or delay cardiac complications and also appears to delay infectious episodes.

In recent years, registry studies have consistently shown a survival benefit of ICT in patients with lower-risk MDS, and these results are now corroborated by an improved EFS demonstrated by the Telesto study. The Kaplan-Meier curves of EFS in the Telesto study separate after 2 years, which is plausible because it takes time for iron-related clinical problems to develop, and therefore also takes time for a clinical benefit of ICT to materialize. Accordingly, patients with transfusion-dependent MDS with a life expectancy of 2 years or more should receive ICT. As the Telesto study included patients with an SF of at least 1000 ng/mL, guidelines using this level of SF as a trigger for initiating ICT are corroborated. It remains an open question whether ICT should be started earlier, given the goal of effective suppression of oxidative stress in patients with IOL. All in all, the Telesto study does not change the hitherto existing recommendations for ICT in patients with MDS. Rather, it helps the believers to justify their use of iron chelators and may lead some nonbelievers to try ICT in some of their transfusion-dependent patients with lower-risk MDS.

REFERENCES

1. Malcovati L, Della Porta MG, Cazzola M. Predicting survival and leukemic evolution in patients with myelodysplastic syndrome. Haematologica 2006;91: 1588–90.

2. de Swart L, Reiniers C, Bagguley T, et al. Labile plasma iron levels predict survival in patients with lower-risk myelodysplastic syndromes. Haematologica 2018;103(1):69–79.

3. Hoeks M, Bagguley T, Roelofs R, et al. Transfusion dependency is associated with presence of toxic iron species and inferior survival in patients with lower-risk myelodysplastic syndromes. 24th European Hematology Association Congress. Amsterdam, June 13-16, 2019. Abstract S838.

4. Carpenter JP, He T, Kirk P, et al. On T2* magnetic resonance and cardiac iron. Circulation 2011;123(14):1519–28.

5. Vinchi F, Muckenthaler MU, Da Silva MC, et al. Atherogenesis and iron: from epidemiology to cellular level. Front Pharmacol 2014;5:94.

6. Duffy SJ, Biegelsen ES, Holbrook M, et al. Iron chelation improves endothelial function in patients with coronary artery disease. Circulation 2001;103(23): 2799–804.

7. Cheung YF, Chan GCF, Ha SY. Effect of deferasirox (ICL670) on arterial function in patients with beta-thalassaemia major. Br J Haematol 2008;141:728–33.

8. Wong CAC, Wong SAY, Leitch HA. Iron overload in lower international prognostic scoring system risk patients with myelodysplastic syndrome receiving red blood cell transfusions: relation to infections and possible benefit of iron chelation therapy. Leuk Res 2018;67:75–81.

9. Leitch HA, Gattermann N. Hematologic improvement with iron chelation therapy in myelodysplastic syndromes: clinical data, potential mechanisms, and outstanding questions. Crit Rev Oncol Hematol 2019;141:54–72.

10. Leitch HA, Parmar A, Wells RA, et al. Overall survival in lower IPSS risk MDS by receipt of iron chelation therapy, adjusting for patient-related factors and measuring from time of first red blood cell transfusion dependence: an MDS-CAN analysis. Br J Haematol 2017;179(1):83–97.

11. Langemeijer S, De Swart L, Yu G, et al. Impact of treatment with iron chelators in lower-risk MDS patients participating in the European Leukemianet MDS (EUMDS) registry. Blood 2016;128:3186.

12. Angelucci E, Li J, Greenberg PL, et al. Safety and efficacy, including event-free survival, of deferasirox versus placebo in iron-overloaded patients with low- and Int-1-Risk Myelodysplastic Syndromes (MDS): outcomes from the random-ized, double-blind Telesto study. Blood 2018;132:234.

13. Wong CAC, Leitch H. Delayed time from RBC transfusion dependence to first post transfusion cardiac event in lower IPSS risk MDS patients receiving iron che-lation therapy. 15th International Symposium on Myelodysplastic Syndromes. Co-penhagen, 2019.

14. Remacha AF, Arrizabalaga B, Villegas A, et al. Evolution of iron overload in pa-tients with low-risk myelodysplastic syndrome: iron chelation therapy and organ complications. Ann Hematol 2015;94(5):779–87.

15. Schetz M, Dasta J, Goldstein S, et al. Drug-induced acute kidney injury. Curr Opin Crit Care 2005;11(6):555–65.

16. Piga A, Fracchia S, Lai ME, et al. Deferasirox effect on renal haemodynamic pa-rameters in patients with transfusion-dependent beta thalassaemia. Br J Haema-tol 2015;168(6):882–90.

17. Meunier M, Ancelet S, Lefebvre C, et al. Reactive oxygen species levels control NF-kappaB activation by low dose deferasirox in erythroid progenitors of low risk myelodysplastic syndromes. Oncotarget 2017;8(62):105510–24.

Assessing Symptom Burden in Myelodysplastic Syndrome/Myeloproliferative Neoplasm Overlap Patients

Juan Garza, MD, Jane Margret Anderson,
Robyn M. Scherber, MD, MPH*

KEYWORDS

- Chronic myelomonocytic leukemia • Chronic neutrophilic leukemia
- Juvenile myelomonocytic leukemia • Atypical chronic myelogenous leukemia
- Symptom burden • Quality of life

KEY POINTS

- Myelodysplastic syndrome/myeloproliferative neoplasm overlap syndromes are rare types of chronic myeloid hematologic neoplasms that present a unique challenge to clinicians owing to the relative rarity of these syndromes.
- Patients with overlap syndrome have similar clinical features, mutations, and disease course, to other chronic myeloid malignancies including myeloproliferative neoplasms and myelodysplastic syndromes.
- It is likely that patients with overlap syndromes experience long standing and at times poorly controlled symptoms that may be underrecognized.
- Overall, symptom burden is an important consideration in patients with overlap syndrome, and efforts are ongoing to further investigate symptom burden in these rare diseases.

INTRODUCTION

The myelodysplastic syndrome/myeloproliferative neoplasm (MDS/MPN) overlap syndromes are a distinct hematologic group classified by the World Health Organization (WHO) and include features of both dysplasia and myeloid cell proliferation. They are a group each with its own defining and distinct features stemming from a stem cell disorder that leads to the combination of cytopenias, dysplasia, and myeloproliferation.

This research did not receive any specific grant from funding agencies in the public, commercial, or not-for-profit sectors.
Department of Hematology and Oncology, Mays Cancer Center at UT Health San Antonio MD Anderson, 7979 Wurzbach Road, San Antonio, TX 78229, USA
* Corresponding author. Department of Hematology and Oncology, Mays Cancer Center at UT Health San Antonio MD Anderson, Urchel Tower #623, 7979 Wurzbach Road, San Antonio, TX 78229, USA.
E-mail address: scherber@uthscsa.edu

Hematol Oncol Clin N Am 34 (2020) 475–489
https://doi.org/10.1016/j.hoc.2019.11.001
0889-8588/20/© 2019 Elsevier Inc. All rights reserved.
hemonc.theclinics.com

Recognized by WHO in 2001, the subtypes included in this category share the common defining feature of their inability to be classified in other specific MDS or MPN disease categories.[1] Included under the umbrella term of MDS/MPN overlap syndrome are: chronic myelomonocytic leukemia (CMML), atypical chronic myeloid leukemia (aCML), juvenile myelomonocytic leukemia (JMML), MDS with ring sideroblasts (MDS-RS), and single lineage dysplasia, previously called refractory anemia with ring sideroblasts (RARS), and the closely related MDS/MPN with ring sideroblasts and thrombocytosis (MDS/MPN-RS-T) formerly known as refractory anemia with ringed sideroblasts and thrombocytosis (RARS-T), and MDS/MPN unclassifiable (MDS/MPN-U).

Although MDS/MPN overlap syndromes are heterogenous and distinct in morphologic and genetic characteristics, they can share strikingly similar clinical manifestations and disease phenotypes. For example, anemia, splenomegaly, abdominal pain, and thrombosis are frequent in all MDS/MPN subtypes. This may be explained by the inflammatory and dysplastic milieu found in the bone marrow within all these subgroups as has been seen in the MPN and MDS disorders.[2] The shared disease phenotypes along with early data regarding symptoms in overlap syndromes suggest that they also share a multifaceted and distinct symptom burden profile, including fatigue, early satiety, abdominal pain and discomfort, and constitutional symptoms. Overlap syndromes also differ in their overall incidence, prognosis and survival, although for all types the incidence is low and survival tends to be worse than many other more common MPN and MDS subtypes. Similar to their MDS and MPN counterparts, certain patient characteristics may lead to a worse prognosis, such as older age of presentation, higher blast count, and blood transfusion dependence.

Our management of MDS/MPN overlap syndromes is primarily anecdotal, as no specific consensus treatment guidelines or randomized prospective trials are available to guide our care in overlap syndromes to date. The treatment foundation continues to be supportive care with cytoreduction therapy and blood transfusions, with allogenic bone marrow transplantation as an early treatment strategy for patients who are eligible. Ongoing clinical trials in overlap syndromes have begun to recognize the importance of symptom burden in this population, and symptom burden assessment has become a primary and secondary endpoint for most of the ongoing and planned clinical trials to date. We have also begun to recognize the importance of symptom assessment, monitoring, and directed therapies in this population. However, these efforts have been limited by the lack of formal published testing and validation of symptom burden profiles in overlap syndromes.

In this article, we aim to detail efforts to date to better understand, assess, and monitor changes of symptom burden in this population. We discuss the specific disease subtype characteristics and clinical features that lead to symptoms, symptom assessment tools that have been used to assess symptoms in patients with overlap syndrome in clinical trials, and the data to date in terms of specific disease symptoms in overlap disease subtypes that have been published to date.

OVERLAP SYNDROMES SUBTYPE DISEASE FEATURES AND SYMPTOMATOLOGY
Chronic Myelomonocytic Leukemia

CMML demonstrates both dysplasia and cytopenias and also has proliferative features, namely in the form of excessive monocytes.[3,4] Prognosis for CMML is variable, and can be separated into 3 broad categories. The first, CMML-0, is characterized by having less than 2% blasts in peripheral blood and less than 5% in bone marrow and has a median overall survival of 32 months. The second, CMML-1, is characterized by less than 5% blasts in peripheral blood and or under 10% blasts in the bone marrow and have a median overall survival of 20 months. The third, CMML-2, has 5% to 19% blasts in peripheral blood and/or 10% to 19% blasts in the bone marrow with a reported median overall survival of 15 months.[5] Elderly patients have the worse survival of approximately 3-year overall survival reported to be 20% and decreasing in those over 80 years of age.[6]

The symptom burden in CMML has been described in at least 1 investigation by Emanuel.[3] The symptoms of fatigue and shortness of breath were significant in this population. Patients also reported common recurrent infections. These symptoms parallel the disease profile, such as anemia, leukocytosis, leukopenia, dysplasia, and thrombocytopenia. Also, splenomegaly has been reported in up to 25% of patients and this may contribute to early satiation, abdominal pain, or discomfort and fatigue.[7]

Atypical Chronic Myeloid Leukemia

aCML is an extremely rare form of leukemia that is classified within myelodysplastic/myeloproliferative diseases according to WHO. Features include neutrophilia with left shift, anemia, thrombocytopenia, and splenomegaly, but patients lack the classic Philadelphia chromosome BCR/ABL translocation.[8] Overall survival is poor and median overall survival has been reported to be about 12 months, with patients transforming to acute myeloid leukemia (AML) within this time frame.[9] Other studies have defined median overall survival to be 14 to 30 months, with a worse prognosis found in those older than 65 years.[10] The symptom burden profile in aCML has not been well defined in studies to date, although clinically it is common that patients complain of splenomegaly related and constitutional symptoms including weight loss, early satiety, and abdominal fullness or pain.[11]

Myelodysplastic Syndrome with Ring Sideroblasts and Myelodysplastic Syndrome/Myeloproliferative Neoplasm with Ring Sideroblasts and Thrombocytosis

MDS-RS and MDS/MPN-RS-T is a relatively new WHO classification entity, with patients presenting with features of MDS-RS and displaying the hyperproliferative feature of thrombocytosis.[8] This is a rare disorder accounting for less than 1% of all MDS cases.[12] The hallmark of this disorder is on one hand the ringed sideroblasts, with iron deposited in the perinuclear mitochondria resulting in sideroblastic anemia, and on the other hand the common SF3B1 mutation with or without JAK2V617 F or other proliferative mutation, such as BCR/ABL1 and PCM1-JAK2 fusion genes, and rearrangement of PDGFRA, PDGFRB, and FGFR1 mutations.[8] Proliferation of megakaryocytes is seen in the bone marrow. Thrombosis risk is also increased because of the nature of thrombocytosis as seen in the closely related essential thrombocythemia.[13] Overall survival has been reported to be about 76 months with variability depending on certain cytogenetic risks and degree of thrombosis.[14]

In 1 study of MDS/MPN-RS-T published by Gurevich and colleagues[15], the presenting signs and symptoms of patients included fatigue (5/18), heavy menstrual bleeding (2/18), epistaxis (2/18), weight loss (1/18), upper respiratory tract infection/flu-like symptoms (2/18), and chest pain (1/18). In this cohort, 5/18 patients presented with incidental findings including anemia and/or thrombocytopenia, but no specific symptoms were reported. Splenomegaly was palpable in 2/18 patients.

Juvenile Myelomonocytic Leukemia

JMML is extremely rare, characterized by dysplastic myelomonocytic cells that infiltrate the bone marrow and even visceral organs.[16] Although this disease is most commonly observed in childhood with a rare incidence of 1.2/million persons in the United States,[16] it can rarely be present in adults. The RAS/MAPK signaling pathway has been seen to be affected in most patients. This results in a signaling pathway that makes it sensitive to monocyte stimulating factors within the bone marrow. Furthermore, mutations in NF1 and PTPN11 are also reported in up to 90% of patients.[17] Congenital disorders, such as Noonan syndrome have been found to have mutations in PTPN11 or RAS in up to half of all patients and are at risk to develop JMML.[18] Median overall survival without transplant has been reported to be 10 to 12 months.[19]

Disease features stem from increased levels of malignant monocytic and myeloid cells in the bone marrow, peripheral blood, and visceral organs. Patients may present with infections, fever, hemorrhage, and fatigue. Also, organomegaly especially splenomegaly and hepatomegaly is observed in up to 95% of all patients.[19] Common clinical symptoms of JMML include pallor, fatigue, weakness, fevers, and a dry cough.[20]

Chronic Neutrophilic Leukemia

Chronic neutrophilic leukemia (CNL) is a rare hematopoietic cell disorder, with a median age at diagnosis of more than 66 years. It consists of an increase in mature granulocyte production. The increased granulocytes infiltrate into visceral organs causing hepatosplenomegaly.[10] WHO criteria for diagnosing CNL requires a white blood cell peripheral blood count above 25K, hypercellular bone marrow, not meeting WHO criteria for BCR-ABL1+ CML, PV, ET, or PMF, no rearrangement of PDGFRA, PDGFRB, FGFR1, or PCM1-JAK2, presence of CSF3R (in the absence of a CSFR3R mutation, persistent neutrophilia [of at least 3 months], splenomegaly, and no identifiable cause of reactive neutrophilia).[8,21] Symptoms of CNL, include fatigue and splenomegaly with some abdominal bloating and satiation. Prognosis continues to be poor and no standard treatment is available although some studies have shown some response to JAK2 inhibitors.[22]

Myelodysplastic Syndrome/Myeloproliferative Neoplasm Unclassifiable

MDS/MPN-U is a disease subtype that has features of both MDS and MPN but does not meet criteria for any of the other subtypes as described above. It is defined as patients with no preceding history of MDS or MPN, without Philadelphia chromosome, BCR-ABL1 fusion gene, PDGFRA, PDGFRB or isolated del(5q), t(3;3) (q21;q26) or inv(3) (q21q26), and less than 20% blasts in the blood and bone marrow, prominent myeloproliferative features, or de novo disease with mixed myeloproliferative and myelodysplastic features that cannot be assigned to any other category of MDS, MPN, or MPS/MPN.[1,23] Common mutations found are ASXL1, TET2, JAK2, and SRSF2, as are SETBP1, DNMT3A, and EZH2 (19%).[24] Further studies have also reported approximately 30% of patients with JAK2-V617 mutation and trisomy 8 in 15% of patients.[23] This subtype is extremely rare and has been described as being lower than 5% of all myeloid neoplasms.[25]

Disease features include splenomegaly in 35% of patients, constitutional symptoms in (69%), leukocytosis greater than 25K (36%) anemia with a hemoglobin count less than 10 (46%), and thrombocytosis greater than 450K in 13% of patients.[23] This subtype is unusual because it is not associated with any particular individual disease feature, and, given the rarity, descriptions of specific symptoms are rare in published findings.

SYMPTOM ORIGIN IN OVERLAP SYNDROMES

Common disease features and characteristics that overlap syndromes shared with MPN and MDS relate back to common etiologies of symptoms in patients with overlap syndrome.[26] The largest and most comprehensive assessment of symptoms to date has been reported in MPN syndromes, with the most prevalent symptoms being fatigue (92.7%), impaired quality of life (84.2%), insomnia (65.4%), sad mood (62.7%), early satiety (61.9%), concentration problems (61.7%), numbness (61.3%), and inactivity (60.5%) (**Fig. 1**).[27] The origins of these symptoms in chronic myeloid diseases can be traced back to disease features including of high/low blood counts, thrombosis, and organ dysfunction, such as splenomegaly and disease progression. Inflammation also plays a key role in terms of symptom development. There is a significant correlation between increased inflammatory cytokines and symptom burden.[2,28–30]

The common molecular pathways including epigenetic dysregulation and excessive JAK1/2 signaling that can be observed in overlap syndromes can stimulate excessive tumor necrosis factor alpha (TNF-α), interleukin-1 (IL-1), and IL-6, and dysregulate B- and T-cell functioning.[31] This understanding of the significance of cytokines in chronic myeloid malignancies has led to the development of therapies that target cytokine levels.[26] Symptoms also occur in the setting of variable baseline health status, with insurance database information suggesting a high rate of Charleston comorbidity indexes among the MDS/MPN overlap disease population, which also can play into worsening of underlying symptomatology. Given the heterogeneity of symptoms, the specific commonly reported symptoms in overlap syndromes and their potential specific etiologies are discussed below.

Fatigue

Fatigue is a common complaint among patients with MDS and MPN syndromes and similarly is commonly reported in patients with CMML and JMML.[3,32,33] Anemia and increased inflammatory cytokines have been reported to play a role in the development of fatigue burden in patients with cancer. Increased TNF-α levels have been shown to be associated with post chemotherapy fatigue in patients with breast cancer.[34] IL-1, IL-6, and TNF-α have also been reported to deregulate erythropoiesis, further exacerbating anemia in patients with AML and MDS.[35]

Abdominal Complaints

Abdominal complaints are common among patients with MPN and MPN/MDS overlap syndrome. Up to 20% to 30% of patients with MPN/MDS have splenomegaly, and in subtypes such as JMML there is an estimated 90% prevalence. Splenomegaly can lead to early satiety, abdominal discomfort, abdominal distension, constipation, and weight loss, as seen in patients with MPN.[27,33] Inflammatory cytokines and inflammation may also play a role in abdominal complaints, because development of splenomegaly has been associated with increased cytokines, such as IL-1 receptor antagonist, and monokine induced by IFN-γ.[36] Also, splenic and portal vein thrombosis may contribute to abdominal pain and discomfort. Patients with MPNs who have a higher C-reactive protein have been reported to have higher rates of major thrombotic events, particularly abdominal vein thrombosis.[37] Because patients with overlap syndromes are reported to have higher rates of thrombosis, especially in MDS/MPN-RS-T and MDS/MPN-U, it is likely that a higher rate of abdominal vein thrombosis is present in this population.

Constitutional Symptoms

Fever, night sweats, and weight loss, collectively known as constitutional symptoms, are commonly seen in patients with MPNs and have also been described in those with

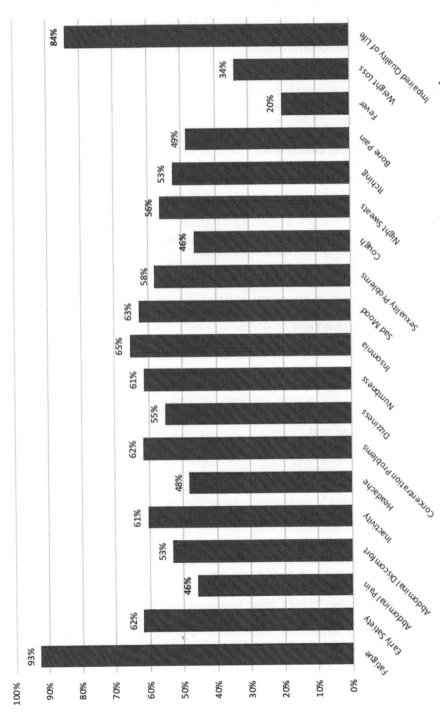

Fig. 1. Common symptoms in MPN patients by prevalence as assessed by the myeloproliferative neoplasm symptom assessment form.

overlap syndrome.[12,23] The role of MPN-associated weight loss has been linked to splenomegaly, cachexia, and portal hypertension, all of which may be seen in the overlap syndromes. Furthermore, inflammatory mediators, such as IL-1, IL-6, and TNF-α have been shown to drive fevers and night sweats. IL-6 has also been found to correlate with B symptoms in patients with chronic lymphocytic leukemia and Hodgkin lymphoma.[38]

Sexual Complaints

Sexual complaints have been reported to be linked to disease and symptom burden in MPNs, and are likely to be present in overlap syndromes also.[28] The overall incidence of sexual complaints is in the 64% range in MPNs. Complaints are correlated with transfusion dependence, severity of cytopenias, and in older patients.[33] Men reported having higher sexual dysfunction symptoms than women. Although not reported in overlap syndrome this may be an unrecognized physiologic and psychological burden in these patients.

Cognitive Complaints

Proinflammatory cytokine production and inflammation occurring at the microvascular level has been thought to lead to symptoms, such as headaches, concentration issues, lightheadedness, vertigo, and even sexual dysfunction. Also, neurocognitive symptoms may be attributed to cellular stasis and microthrombosis.[2] Increased levels of IL-6 have been shown to correlate in human subjects with impaired memory and learning.[39] Patients with hematologic disorders and increased IL-6 levels have been reported to have worsened executive function.[35] This may well apply to overlap syndrome because it too has increased levels of inflammation.

Depression

Depression has been reported to occur in all cancer types and is related to the degree of symptom burden. Up to 30% of patients with MPN have been reported to have depression, and this may reflect or parallel that seen in patients with overlap syndromes. Fatigue, sexual dysfunction, and pain have all been related to the increasing levels of depression seen in patients with cancer. IL-6 has also been reported to be associated with depression and fatigue in patients with MPNs accounting for a systemic inflammatory milieu.[38] Sedentary lifestyle may also exacerbate a proinflammatory state and further lead to more depression.

ASSESSING SYMPTOM BURDEN IN OVERLAP SYNDROMES

Because MPN/MDS overlap syndromes have characteristics of both MPN and MDS, many of the symptom tools utilized to date to assess symptoms in patients with overlap syndrome have been designed for use in more common but closely related MPNs, MDS, and in other hematologic malignancies. Specifically, the Myeloproliferative Neoplasm Symptom Assessment Form (MPN-SAF), Myeloproliferative Neoplasm Symptom Assessment Form Total Symptom Score (MPN-SAF TSS or MPN-10), EQ-5D, European Organization for Research and Treatment of Cancer (EORTC), Functional Assessment of Cancer Therapy-Leukemia (FACT-Leu), and Functional Assessment of Cancer Therapy-Anemia (FACT-An) have all been utilized in clinical trials or have rationale use to assess symptom burden in patients with overlap syndrome (**Table 1**). These patient-reported outcome (PRO) tools have aided in assessing the benefits of therapies but have not been validated in this population. Below, we discuss the available specific symptom assessment tools that have rationale use in the overlap syndromes.

Table 1
Variables utilized in the symptom assessment tools with rationale use in patients with overlap syndrome

	Fatigue	Abdominal Complaints	Sexual Complaints	Cognitive Complaints	Mood/ Depression	Overall Pain
MPN-SAF	O	O	O	O	O	
MPN-10	O	O		O		
EQ-5D					O	O
EORTC	O	O		O	O	O
FACT-Leu	O	O	O		O	O
FACT-An	O	O	O		O	O

Myeloproliferative Neoplasm Symptom Assessment Form

The MPN-SAF is a 27-item PRO that has been validated for the assessment of symptom burden in myeloproliferative neoplasms.[33] MPN-SAF is the largest assessment of symptom burden of MPN patients to date and has been validated in over 2000 patients internationally, as well as translated into over 11 languages. Studies showed the MPN-SAF scores were in concordance with the EORTC QLQ-C30.[33] The scale for the MPN-SAF ranges from 0 (absent) to 10 (worst imaginable) for 17 items including fatigue (utilizing the brief fatigue inventory), early satiety, abdominal pain, abdominal discomfort, inactivity, cough, night sweats, pruritus, bone pain, fever, weight loss, overall quality of life, headaches, concentration, dizziness/vertigo/lightheadedness, numbness/tingling, sleeping difficulties, mood, and sexual function.[33]

Myeloproliferative Neoplasm Symptom Assessment Form Total Symptom Score

The MPN-SAF TSS (also known as MPN-10) measure consists of 10 questions focusing on fatigue, concentration, early satiety, inactivity, night sweats, itching, bone pain, abdominal discomfort, weight loss, and fevers.[30] The MPN-10 scale ranges from 0 (absent) to 10 (worst imaginable) and the items assessed through the MPN-10 can be looked at individually or summed for the total symptom score. Individual symptom scores are added together to calculate a TSS with higher scores representing worse symptom burden and functions. The total symptom score ranges from 0 to 100. The MPN-10 has been validated in myeloproliferative neoplasms and is the most widely utilized to date of the MPN symptom assessments in clinical trials.[27,40]

EQ-5D

The EQ-5D was developed by the European Quality of Life Group and can be used to measure quality of life in a variety of health conditions. There are currently 3 versions of the EQ-5D: one with 3 levels of severity for 5 dimensions (EQ-5D-3 L), one with 5 levels of severity for each of the 5 dimensions (EQ-5D-3 L), and one for children (EQ-5D-Y). The 5 dimensions included in the descriptive system are mobility, self-care, usual activities, pain/discomfort, and anxiety/depression. In addition to the descriptive system, the EQ-5D also contains the EQ visual analogue scale (VAS). The EQ VAS measures the patient's self-rated health on a vertical VAS reflecting the patient's judgment. Although we did not see significant validation for EQ-5D in overlap syndromes, the National Institute for Health and Care Excellence (United Kingdom) recommends that a study be conducted evaluating EQ-5D values in patients with MDS, CMML, or AML.

European Organization for Research and Treatment of Cancer QLQ-C30

The EORTC QLQ-C30 is made up of 30 items covering 5 functional scales, 9 symptom scales, and a global health status/quality of life scale. Twenty-eight of the questions have 4 responses (not at all, a little, quite a bit, and very much). Two of the 30 questions have a 7-point rating scale. The raw score is converted into scores ranging from 0 to 100 with a higher score representing a better quality of life. The EORTC QLQ-C30 was validated in 1997 in patients with cancer.[41]

Functional Assessment of Cancer Therapy: Leukemia

FACT-Leu was developed for patients with acute and chronic leukemia. The FACT-Leu version 5.0 is a 44-item questionnaire with answers ranging from 0 (not at all) to 4 (very much). A meaningful clinical change in the FACT-Leu is a 13- to 17-point difference.[42] The FACT-Leu was validated in 79 patients with acute or chronic leukemia in 2012.[43]

Functional Assessment of Cancer Therapy: Anemia

FACT-An is a 48-item PRO and has been tested for reliability, validity, and responsiveness in MDS patients who are low or Int-1 risk with del5q.[44] Like FACT-Leu, it uses a scale ranging from 0 (not at all) to 4 (very much). FACT-An might be a significant quality of life assessment tool in overlap syndromes because of the large role anemia plays in symptom burden.

SYMPTOM ASSESSMENT IN SPECIFIC OVERLAP SUBTYPES

Clinical trials looking at overlap syndromes have used various symptom assessment tools to assess therapeutic benefit including the MPN-10, MPN-SAF, EORTC, FACT-Leu, and FACT-An; however, there remains a general paucity of available published studies in regard to symptom burden in overlap syndromes. In our search of the use of symptom assessment forms in overlap syndromes, we found no validation of a symptom assessment tool and only found use of symptom assessment tools in clinical trials (**Table 2**).

Symptom Assessment in Chronic Myelomonocytic Leukemia

The symptom burden in CMML has been assessed via MPN-10, MPN-SAF, EORTC, FACT-Leu, and FACT-An. Historically, therapeutic response in CMML patients has been measured via the International Working Group (IWG) response criteria for MDS.[45] However, more recently, PROs have been used to assess therapeutic benefit. MPN-10 was used in a clinical trial assessing ruxolitinib for the treatment of CMML in a phase 2 expansion through rankings of 0 (symptom is absent) to 10 (worst imaginable) (NCT03722407[46]). MPN-SAF and EORTC were both used to evaluate the quality of life and patient-reported symptoms in CMML patients treated with LDE224 in addition to azacitidine or decitabine (NCT02129101[47]). Therapeutic responses in CMML have also been measured using EORTC in 4 other clinical trials (NCT03268954[48] NCT01241500[49] NCT01928537[50] and NCT00043134[51]). Finally, FACT-Leu (NCT02749708[52]) and FACT-An (NCT02891551[53] and NCT00274820[54]) have been used to assess therapeutic benefits in CMML.

Symptom Burden Assessment in Chronic Neutrophilic Leukemia and Atypical Chronic Myeloid Leukemia

Symptom burden in aCML and CNL has been assessed via MPN-10. MPN-10 was used in a clinical trial assessing ruxolitinib phosphate in patients with CNL and aCML to

Table 2
Variables utilized in the symptom assessment tools with rationale use in patients with overlap syndrome

Scale Used	Interventions	Study N/Design	Source
CMML			
MPN-10	Ruxolitinib	Phase 2 trial n = 29	NCT03722407
MPN-SAF	LDE225 with azacitidine or decitabine	Phase 1 trial n = 78	NCT02129101
EORTC QLQ-C30	LDE225 with azacitidine or decitabine	Phase 1 trial n = 78	NCT02129101
	Azacitidine and pevonedistat vs azacitidine	Phase 3 trial n = 450	NCT03268954
	ON 01910.Na	Phase 3 trial n = 299	NCT01241500
	Rigosertib sodium	Phase 3 trial n = 67	NCT01928537
	Decitabine	Randomized Clinical Trial- Phase 3 n = 220	NCT00043134 Abstract: Lubbert et al 2011
FACT-Leu	IRX5183	Phase 1 trial[a] n = 13	NCT02749708
FACT-An	Noninterventional. All patients started on azacitidine before initiation	n = 150	NCT02891551
	Thalidomide, arsenic trioxide, dexamethasone, and ascorbic acid (TADA)	Phase 2 trial n = 15	NCT00274820
aCML			
MPN-10	Ruxolitinib phosphate	Phase 2 trial n = 50	NCT02092324 Abstract: Dao et al. 2018
CNL			
MPN-10	Ruxolitinib phosphate	Phase 2 trial n = 50	NCT02092324 Abstract: Dao et al. 2018
MPN/MDS unspecified			
MPN-10	Pacritinib and decitabine	Phase 1 [a]n = 0	NCT02564536

[a] Withdrawn or terminated.

determine the mean percent reduction of total symptom score (NCT02092324[55]). Dao and colleagues found a mean symptom score reduction of 21% by the end of cycle 2 and a 42% reduction by the end of cycle 6 after administration of ruxolitinib phosphate.[56] Despite the use of symptom burden assessment tools in clinical trials, they have not been validated in patients with overlap and there is no uniformly accepted assessment tool for this patient population.

FUTURE ENDEAVORS IN OVERLAP SYNDROME SYMPTOM BURDEN ASSESSMENTS

The robust data in MPNs in regard to the importance of symptom burden for disease monitoring, outcomes, and prognosis, and the growing evidence of the relationship between symptom burden and disease inflammation and other biological markers initially sparked interest in the development of a specific symptom assessment tool specific to overlap syndromes. In 2015, response criteria were developed by an international consortium. This panel recommended that the use of the MPN-10/TSS provides the best potential for symptom assessment and recommended that the commonly used threshold of requiring a 50% reduction to equate a clinical benefit chosen to be consistent with both IWG-MRT/ELN criteria in MPN. More recently, Padron and colleagues, noted that patients with CMML undergoing ruxolitinib treatment reported a dramatic improvement in fatigue and B symptoms based on abstraction of medical records and investigator interview; however, patient-reported FACT-Leu and EORTC QLQ-C30 scales did not seem to adequately capture this change. The investigators suggested that this discrepancy is explained by either an overestimation of effect detailed in the medical record or a lack of sensitivity of the tested scales to measure the improvement in symptoms, both a result of the lack of validation of these tools in CMML.[52] Given this and the potential unique symptom profile in these patients, efforts are underway to design a unique overlap symptom assessment tool to be developed to accurately depict symptom burden in these patients.[26] Currently, efforts are underway to create a validated symptom assessment tool in MDS/MPN (R.A. Mesa, personal communication, 2019).[45] In the meantime, the MPN-10 has been adopted by some centers for clinical symptom monitoring in patients with MPN and has been the most frequently included symptom burden assessment in overlap syndrome clinical trials.

SUMMARY

MDS/MPN overlap syndromes have a unique and diverse symptom burden that at times can be underrecognized. Patients with these chronic myeloid diseases can have indolent disease courses that often will leave patients with decreased quality of life. Symptoms including fatigue, abdominal pain, early satiety, and weight loss have been reported individually in overlap syndrome subtypes. These symptoms likely stem from the underlying disease processes including splenomegaly, blood count abnormalities, thrombosis, and inflammatory cytokines. With the advent of many future pharmacologic therapies that may decrease symptom burden, efforts to further quantify and objectively assess symptom burden both initially at diagnosis and over the course of pharmacologic interventions are necessary and essential to help optimize patient outcomes and functioning. Many clinical trials already incorporate symptom burden assessments in trials, and early data suggest that a tailored symptom burden assessment tool, such as the MPN-10, or even a tool developed specifically for overlap syndromes, may represent the optimal symptom assessment method. Efforts are ongoing to better understand, assess, and monitor symptom burden in these unique and rare myeloid malignancies.

REFERENCES

1. Vardiman JW, Thiele J, Arber DA, et al. The 2008 revision of the World Health Organization (WHO) classification of myeloid neoplasms and acute leukemia: rationale and important changes. Blood 2009;114(5):937–51. Available at: https://www.ncbi.nlm.nih.gov/pubmed/19357394.
2. Geyer HL, Dueck AC, Scherber RM, et al. Impact of inflammation on myeloproliferative neoplasm symptom development. Mediators Inflamm 2015;2015:284706.
3. Emanuel PD. Juvenile myelomonocytic leukemia and chronic myelomonocytic leukemia. Leukemia 2008;22(7):1335–42.

4. Germing U, Gattermann N, Minning H, et al. Problems in the classification of CMML-dysplastic versus proliferative type. Leuk Res 1998;22(10):871–8. Available at: https://www.sciencedirect.com/science/article/abs/pii/S01452126970 01926?via%3Dihub.

5. Germing U, Kündgen A, Gattermann N. Risk assessment in chronic myelomonocytic leukemia (CMML). Leuk Lymphoma 2004;45(7):1311–8.

6. Rollison DE, Howlader N, Smith MT, et al. Epidemiology of myelodysplastic syndromes and chronic myeloproliferative disorders in the United States, 2001–2004, using data from the NAACCR and SEER programs. Blood 2008;112(1):45–52. Available at: https://www.ncbi.nlm.nih.gov/pubmed/18443215.

7. Kantarjian H, Oki Y, Garcia-Manero G, et al. Results of a randomized study of 3 schedules of low-dose decitabine in higher-risk myelodysplastic syndrome and chronic myelomonocytic leukemia. Blood 2007;109(1):52–7. Available at: https://www.ncbi.nlm.nih.gov/pubmed/16882708.

8. Arber DA, Orazi A, Hasserjian R, et al. The 2016 revision to the World Health Organization classification of myeloid neoplasms and acute leukemia. Blood 2016; 127(20):2391–405. Available at: https://www.ncbi.nlm.nih.gov/pubmed/27069254.

9. Wang SA, Hasserjian RP, Fox PS, et al. Atypical chronic myeloid leukemia is clinically distinct from unclassifiable myelodysplastic/myeloproliferative neoplasms. Blood 2014;123(17):2645–51. Available at: https://www.ncbi.nlm.nih.gov/pubmed/24627528.

10. Gotlib J, Maxson JE, George TI, et al. The new genetics of chronic neutrophilic leukemia and atypical CML: implications for diagnosis and treatment. Blood 2013;122(10):1707–11. Available at: https://www.ncbi.nlm.nih.gov/pubmed/23896413.

11. Dao KT, Tyner JW. What's different about atypical CML and chronic neutrophilic leukemia? Hematology Am Soc Hematol Educ Program 2015;2015(1):264–71. Available at: https://www.ncbi.nlm.nih.gov/pubmed/26637732.

12. Orazi A, Germing U. The myelodysplastic/myeloproliferative neoplasms: myeloproliferative diseases with dysplastic features. Leukemia 2008;22:1308–19.

13. Patnaik MM, Tefferi A. Refractory anemia with ring sideroblasts (RARS) and RARS with thrombocytosis (RARS-T): 2017 update on diagnosis, risk-stratification, and management. Am J Hematol 2017;92(3):297–310. Available at: https://onlinelibrary.wiley.com/doi/abs/10.1002/ajh.24637.

14. Gattermann N, Billiet J, Kronenwett R, et al. High frequency of the JAK2 V617F mutation in patients with thrombocytosis (platelet count > 600 x 109/L) and ringed sideroblasts more than 15% considered as MDS/MPD, unclassifiable. Blood 2007; 109(3):1334–5. Available at: https://www.ncbi.nlm.nih.gov/pubmed/17244688.

15. Gurevich I, Luthra R, Konoplev SN, et al. Refractory anemia with ring sideroblasts associated with marked thrombocytosis: a mixed group exhibiting a spectrum of morphologic findings. Am J Clin Pathol 2011;135(3):398–403.

16. Chan RJ, Cooper T, Kratz CP, et al. Juvenile myelomonocytic leukemia: a report from the 2nd International JMML Symposium. Leuk Res 2008;33(3):355–62. Available at: https://www.clinicalkey.es/playcontent/1-s2.0-S0145212608003767.

17. Loh ML. Recent advances in the pathogenesis and treatment of juvenile myelomonocytic leukaemia. Br J Haematol 2011;152(6):677.

18. Ekvall S, Wilbe M, Dahlgren J, et al. Mutation in NRAS in familial Noonan syndrome—case report and review of the literature. BMC Med Genet 2015;16(1):95. Available at: https://www.ncbi.nlm.nih.gov/pubmed/26467218.

19. Niemeyer CM, Arico M, Basso G, et al. Chronic myelomonocytic leukemia in childhood: a retrospective analysis of 110 cases. European working group on

myelodysplastic syndromes in childhood (EWOG-MDS). Blood 1997;89(10): 3534–43. Available at: https://www.ncbi.nlm.nih.gov/pubmed/9160658.

20. Juvenile myelomonocytic leukemia. National Organization for Rare Disorders Web site. Available at: https://rarediseases.org/rare-diseases/juvenile-myelomonocytic-leukemia/.

21. Maxson JE, Gotlib J, Pollyea DA, et al. Oncogenic CSF3R mutations in chronic neutrophilic leukemia and atypical CML. N Engl J Med 2013;368(19):1781–90.

22. Elliott MA, Tefferi A. Chronic neutrophilic leukemia 2018: update on diagnosis, molecular genetics, prognosis, and management. Am J Hematol 2018;93:578–87.

23. Dinardo CD, Daver N, Jain N, et al. Myelodysplastic/myeloproliferative neoplasms, unclassifiable (MDS/MPN, U): natural history and clinical outcome by treatment strategy. Leukemia 2014;28(4):958–61. Available at: https://www.ncbi.nlm.nih.gov/pubmed/24492324.

24. Hendrix K, Alali N, Padron E, et al. Myelodysplastic/myeloproliferative neoplasms unclassified (MDS/MPN-U) overlap: can we alter the natural history? Blood 2016; 128(22):3125.

25. Cannella L, Breccia M, Latagliata R, et al. Clinical and prognostic features of patients with myelodysplastic/myeloproliferative syndrome categorized as unclassified (MDS/MPD-U) by WHO classification. Leuk Res 2008;32(3):514.

26. Mughal TI, Cross NCP, Padron E, et al. An international MDS/MPN working group's perspective and recommendations on molecular pathogenesis, diagnosis and clinical characterization of myelodysplastic/myeloproliferative neoplasms. Haematologica 2015;100(9):1117–30. Available at: https://www.ncbi.nlm.nih.gov/pubmed/26341525.

27. Scherber R, Dueck A, Kiladjian J, et al. The myeloproliferative neoplasm symptom assessment from (MPN-SAF) derived total symptom score (TSS): an international trial of 1433 patients with myeloproliferative neoplasms (MPNs). Blood 2011; 118(21):3839. Available at: http://www.bloodjournal.org/content/118/21/3839.

28. Geyer HL, Dueck AC, Emanuel RM, et al. Sexuality challenges, intimacy, and MPN symptom burden: An analysis by the MPN quality of life international study group (MPN-QOL ISG). Blood 2013;122(21):4088.

29. Bower JE, Ganz PA, Desmond KA, et al. Fatigue in long-term breast carcinoma survivors: a longitudinal investigation. Cancer 2006;106(4):751–8. Available at: https://www.ncbi.nlm.nih.gov/pubmed/16400678.

30. Emanuel RM, Dueck AC, Geyer HL, et al. Myeloproliferative neoplasm (MPN) symptom assessment form total symptom score: prospective international assessment of an abbreviated symptom burden scoring system among patients with MPNs. J Clin Oncol 2012;30(33):4098–103. Available at: http://jco.ascopubs.org/content/30/33/4098.abstract.

31. Sochacki AL, Fischer MA, Savona MR. Therapeutic approaches in myelofibrosis and myelodysplastic/myeloproliferative overlap syndromes. Onco Targets Ther 2016;2016(Issue 1):2273–86. Available at: https://doaj.org/article/de39f3c1704d43bdbb89b831484aa5c5.

32. Mesa RA, Schwager S, Radia D, et al. The myelofibrosis symptom assessment form (MFSAF): an evidence-based brief inventory to measure quality of life and symptomatic response to treatment in myelofibrosis. Leuk Res 2009;33(9): 1199–203. Available at: https://www.clinicalkey.es/playcontent/1-s2.0-S0145212609000054X.

33. Scherber R, Dueck AC, Johansson P, et al. The myeloproliferative neoplasm symptom assessment form (MPN-SAF): international prospective validation and

reliability trial in 402 patients. Blood 2011;118(2):401–8. Available at: https://www.ncbi.nlm.nih.gov/pubmed/21536863.

34. Bower JE, Ganz PA, Irwin MR, et al. Inflammation and behavioral symptoms after breast cancer treatment: do fatigue, depression, and sleep disturbance share a common underlying mechanism? J Clin Oncol 2011;29(26):3517–22. Available at: http://jco.ascopubs.org/content/29/26/3517.abstract.

35. Meyers CA, Albitar M, Estey E. Cognitive impairment, fatigue, and cytokine levels in patients with acute myelogenous leukemia or myelodysplastic syndrome. Cancer 2005;104(4):788–93.

36. Ayalew T, Vaidya R, Caramazza D, et al. Circulating interleukin (IL)-8, IL-2R, IL-12, and IL-15 levels are independently prognostic in primary myelofibrosis: a comprehensive cytokine profiling study. J Clin Oncol 2011;29(10):1356–63. Available at: http://jco.ascopubs.org/content/29/10/1356.abstract.

37. Barbui T, Carobbio A, Guido F, et al. Inflammation and thrombosis in essential thrombocythemia and polycythemia vera: different role of C-reactive protein and pentraxin 3. Haematologica 2011;96(2):315–8. Available at: http://www.haematologica.org/content/96/2/315.abstract.

38. Seymour JF, Talpaz M, Cabanillas F, et al. Serum interleukin-6 levels correlate with prognosis in diffuse large-cell lymphoma. J Clin Oncol 1995;13(3):575–82.

39. Sparkman NL, Buchanan JB, Heyen JRR, et al. Interleukin-6 facilitates lipopolysaccharide-induced disruption in working memory and expression of other proinflammatory cytokines in hippocampal neuronal cell layers. J Neurosci 2006;26(42):10709–16. Available at: http://www.jneurosci.org/cgi/content/abstract/26/42/10709.

40. Altomare I, Gerds AT, Lessen D, et al. Correlation between MPN-SAF TSS and EORTC QLQ-C30 scores in patients with PV: data from the reveal study. Blood 2018;132(Suppl 1):2259. Available at: http://www.bloodjournal.org/content/132/Suppl_1/2259.

41. Groenvold M, Klee MC, Sprangers MAG, et al. Validation of the EORTC QLQ-C30 quality of life questionnaire through combined qualitative and quantitative assessment of patient-observer agreement. J Clin Epidemiol 1997;50(4):441–50.

42. Bryant AL, Gosselin T, Coffman EM, et al. Symptoms, mobility and function, and quality of life in adults with acute leukemia during initial hospitalization. Oncol Nurs Forum 2018;45(5):653.

43. Cella D, Jensen SE, Webster K, et al. Measuring health-related quality of life in leukemia: the functional assessment of cancer therapy—leukemia (FACT-leu) questionnaire. Value Health 2012;15(8):1051–8. Available at: https://www.clinicalkey.es/playcontent/1-s2.0-S1098301512039320.

44. Brandenburg NA, Yu R, Revicki DA. Reliability and validity of the FACT-an in patients with low or int-1-risk myelodysplastic syndromes with deletion 5q. Blood 2010;116(21):3827. Available at: http://www.bloodjournal.org/content/116/21/3827.

45. Savona MR, Malcovati L, Komrokji R, et al. An international consortium proposal of uniform response criteria for myelodysplastic/myeloproliferative neoplasms (MDS/MPN) in adults. Blood 2015;125(12):1857–65. Available at: https://www.ncbi.nlm.nih.gov/pubmed/25624319.

46. Ruxolitinib for the treatment of chronic myelomonocytic leukemia (CMML): a phase 2 expansion status: recruiting. Available at: https://ClinicalTrials.gov/show/NCT03722407.

47. Azacitidine and sonidegib or decitabine in treating patients with myeloid malignancies status: active, not recruiting. Available at: https://ClinicalTrials.gov/show/NCT02129101.
48. Pevonedistat plus azacitidine versus single-agent azacitidine as first-line treatment for participants with higher-risk myelodysplastic syndromes (HR MDS), chronic myelomonocytic leukemia (CMML), or low-blast acute myelogenous leukemia (AML) status: recruiting. Available at: https://ClinicalTrials.gov/show/NCT03268954.
49. Randomized study of ON 01910.na in refractory myelodysplastic syndrome patients with excess blasts status: active, not recruiting. Available at: https://ClinicalTrials.gov/show/NCT01241500.
50. Efficacy and safety of IV rigosertib in MDS patients with excess blasts progressing after azacitidine or decitabine status: active, not recruiting. Available at: https://ClinicalTrials.gov/show/NCT01928537.
51. Low-dose decitabine compared with standard supportive care in treating older patients with myelodysplastic syndrome status: unknown status. Available at: https://ClinicalTrials.gov/show/NCT00043134.
52. Study of IRX5183 in relapsed and refractory acute myeloid leukemia and high risk myelodysplastic syndrome status: terminated. Available at: https://ClinicalTrials.gov/show/NCT02749708.
53. An observational post authorisation study to evaluate safety and efficacy in patients receiving azacitidine in daily clinical practice in the Netherlands status: completed. Available at: https://ClinicalTrials.gov/show/NCT02891551.
54. Arsenic trioxide, ascorbic acid, dexamethasone, and thalidomide in myelofibrosis/myeloproliferative disorder status: completed. Available at: https://ClinicalTrials.gov/show/NCT00274820.
55. Ruxolitinib phosphate in treating patients with chronic neutrophilic leukemia or atypical chronic myeloid leukemia status: recruiting. Available at: https://ClinicalTrials.gov/show/NCT02092324.
56. Dao K, Collins RH, Cortes JE, et al. Phase 2 Study of Ruxolitinib in Patients with Chronic Neutrophilic Leukemia or Atypical Chronic Myeloid Leukemia. Blood 2018;132(Suppl 1):350.

Moving?

Make sure your subscription moves with you!

To notify us of your new address, find your **Clinics Account Number** (located on your mailing label above your name), and contact customer service at:

Email: journalscustomerservice-usa@elsevier.com

800-654-2452 (subscribers in the U.S. & Canada)
314-447-8871 (subscribers outside of the U.S. & Canada)

Fax number: 314-447-8029

Elsevier Health Sciences Division
Subscription Customer Service
3251 Riverport Lane
Maryland Heights, MO 63043